CRAM SESSION IN

General Medical Conditions

A Handbook for Students & Clinicians

ROBB S. REHBERG ▪ JOELLE STABILE REHBERG

CRAM SESSION IN
General Medical Conditions

A Handbook for Students & Clinicians

ROBB S. REHBERG ▪ JOELLE STABILE REHBERG

ROBB S. REHBERG, PHD, ATC, NREMT
William Paterson University
Wayne, New Jersey

JOELLE STABILE REHBERG, DO
Atlantic Neurosurgical Specialists
Morristown, New Jersey

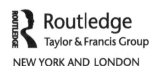

Routledge
Taylor & Francis Group

NEW YORK AND LONDON

Robb S. Rehberg, PhD, ATC, NREMT and Joelle Stabile Rehberg, DO have no financial or proprietary interest in the materials presented herein.

First published in 2012 by SLACK Incorporated

Published in 2024 by Routledge
605 Third Avenue, New York, NY 10158

and by Routledge
4 Park Square, Milton Park, Abingdon, Oxon, OX14 4RN

Routledge is an imprint of the Taylor & Francis Group, an informa business

Rehberg, Robb S.
  Cram session in general medical conditions : a handbook for students and clinicians / Robb S. Rehberg, Joelle Stabile Rehberg.
      p. ; cm.
  Includes bibliographical references and index.
  ISBN 9781556429484 (pbk. : alk. paper)
  I. Rehberg, Joelle Stabile. II. Title.
  [DNLM: 1. Clinical Medicine--Handbooks. 2. Disease--Handbooks. WB 39]
  L Cclassification not assigned
  616--dc23
                          2012002880

ISBN: 9781556429484 (pbk)
ISBN: 9781003523406 (ebk)

DOI: 10.4324/9781003523406

DEDICATION

To Anna and Joey, for waiting patiently while Mommy and Daddy finished their "homework" (this book). You are the light of our lives.

And for our parents, Bert and Lynda Rehberg, and Jeff and Maryann Stabile.

CONTENTS

ACKNOWLEDGMENTS

The authors would like to thank the following individuals whose research assistance was essential to the development of this book:

John Patrick Acosta, ATC
Taylor Alda, ATC
Nicole Callaghan, ATC
Golam Chowdhury, EMT
Monique Gerald, ATC
Michael Prybicien, MA, ATC
Justin Schmarak

ABOUT THE AUTHORS

Robb S. Rehberg, PhD, ATC, NREMT is an associate professor and coordinator of athletic training clinical education at William Paterson University in Wayne, New Jersey. He also serves as an athletic trainer for Atlantic Health System/Overlook Medical Center in Summit, New Jersey, and is a founding partner of The Rehberg Konin Group. He also served as the Director and Chief of Emergency Services at Montclair State University in Montclair, New Jersey from 1998 to 2010. Prior to teaching at William Paterson, Dr. Rehberg spent 13 years as the head athletic trainer at Westwood Regional High School in Westwood, New Jersey. Dr. Rehberg earned his doctorate (PhD) in Health Science from Touro University International in 2003, a master of sport science (MSS) degree from the United States Sports Academy in 1999; and a bachelor of science (BS) degree in Athletic Training from West Chester University in 1991. Dr. Rehberg has spent his career working in both the athletic training and emergency services fields and has published and spoken frequently at state and national meetings on sports emergency care. Dr. Rehberg served as a member of the medical staff for athletics (track and field) at the 1996 Olympic Games in Atlanta, Georgia. He is active on the state and national level, and currently serves on the National Athletic Trainers' Association (NATA) Research and Education Foundation's Board of Directors. He has also served on the Inter-Association Task Force for the Appropriate Care of the Spine-Injured Athlete, the Task Force on Appropriate Medical Coverage for the Secondary School-Aged Athlete, and the NATA Hall of Fame subcommittee. Dr. Rehberg currently serves as Past-President and coordinator of Governmental Relations for the Athletic Trainers' Society of New Jersey and as the chair of the National Safety Council Emergency Care Advisory Committee. He was a member of the American Heart Association Task Force that developed the first international guidelines for first aid in 2000. He is a charter member of the New Jersey Disaster Medical Assistance Team.

Joelle Stabile Rehberg, DO is a sports medicine-trained primary care physician practicing sports medicine, spine, and concussion management with Atlantic Neurosurgical Specialists in Morristown, New Jersey. Dr. Rehberg also practices at the Center for Concussion Care and Physical Rehabilitation at Atlantic Health System/Overlook Medical Center in Summit, New Jersey. Dr. Rehberg has served as the team physician for Montville High School in Montville, New Jersey, for the past 10 years. She also serves as the medical director for the Athletic Training Education Program at William Paterson University, a post she has held since 2001. Dr. Rehberg graduated from the University of Medicine and Dentistry of New Jersey School of Osteopathic Medicine in 1997. She completed her undergraduate studies in 1993 at Seton Hall University.

PREFACE

There are, perhaps, as many symptoms of human disease as there are colors in the spectrum. And just as a picture is defined by its colors, disease is defined by its collective symptoms. For instance, imagine a painting of a beautiful sunset over a beach. Think of all the shades of color used to paint the picture—different hues of yellow, orange, and red emanating from a setting sun in a bright blue sky shining over a sea of green. White spray from crashing waves lands on a sandy brown beach. We are able to understand exactly what this picture portrays because of the many colors involved. It would be difficult—if not impossible—to interpret the painting if it was painted in only one color. The more shades of color used to paint the picture, the more vivid and clear the picture becomes. The same can be said for recognizing and diagnosing illness. Think of each symptom as a color. The more symptoms that are revealed, the more definitive the diagnosis becomes.

There are many conditions listed in this book that share similar symptoms. Take pain, for instance. If pain was the only symptom revealed while evaluating a patient, it would be difficult, if not impossible, to reach a conclusive diagnosis. The key to effective assessment is uncovering the collections and combinations of symptoms that present through a thorough history and physical exam.

The idea is simple—the more colors, the more clear the picture. The more symptoms recognized, the more definitive the diagnosis.

This book was developed with both the student and the practitioner in mind. It is intended to serve as a refresher on the basics of general medical conditions, providing the quick and useful information necessary to understand each condition, especially those that may not be seen every day. This book is not intended to be a definitive encyclopedia of medical conditions. There are several other excellent textbooks that can provide comprehensive information on general medical conditions, and the authors strongly encourage readers to seek additional information for conditions with which they are unfamiliar. Rather, students may find this book useful as a primer or as a study guide for general medical conditions, while practicing clinicians may find it a handy quick reference guide or refresher that can be useful when presented with conditions they do not commonly encounter.

1

CARDIOVASCULAR CONDITIONS

- ☐ Angina pectoris
- ☐ Atrial fibrillation
- ☐ Coronary artery disease
- ☐ Deep vein thrombosis
- ☐ Dyslipidemia
- ☐ Hypertension
- ☐ Hypotension
- ☐ Myocardial infarction
- ☐ Palpitations
- ☐ Peripheral arterial disease
- ☐ Shock
- ☐ Supraventricular tachycardia
- ☐ Ventricular fibrillation
- ☐ Ventricular tachycardia

Rehberg RS, Rehberg JS.
Cram Session in General Medical Conditions:
A Handbook for Students & Clinicians (pp. 1-18).
© 2012 Taylor & Francis Group.

ANGINA PECTORIS

- ☐ Also known as: Angina

- ☐ Description: Chest discomfort associated with myocardial ischemia and left ventricular dysfunction. Angina is the most common clinical manifestation of coronary artery disease (CAD). Angina that has remained unchanged for 60 days is considered stable angina. Angina that increases in frequency, lasts longer, or is provoked by less exertion is considered unstable angina.

- ☐ Causes

  - ○ Anemia

  - ○ Valvular heart disease

  - ○ Hyperthyroidism

- ☐ Risk factors

  - ○ Hypertension

  - ○ Dyslipidemia

  - ○ Diabetes mellitus

  - ○ Family history of CAD

  - ○ Smoking

- ☐ Clinical presentation

  - ○ Chest pressure

  - ○ Chest tightness and heaviness brought on by exercise or emotional stress

  - ○ Symptoms resolve at rest or upon administration of sublingual nitroglycerin

- ☐ Diagnosis: Electrocardiogram (EKG) and stress testing. Cardiac enzyme blood tests rule out myocardial infarction.

- ☐ Management: Long-acting nitrates, beta-blockers, calcium-channel blockers, and aspirin are commonly used in combination to control symptoms. Percutaneous coronary angioplasty and coronary artery bypass graft (CABG) surgery are considered if symptoms continue despite medical treatment. Correction of underlying conditions and reduction of risk factors are important for managing angina.

ATRIAL FIBRILLATION

- Also known as: A-fib, auricular fibrillation

- Description: Atrial fibrillation occurs when the atria of the heart fibrillates; in other words, there is a twitching of the heart muscle that causes an arrhythmia (irregular heart beat). The heart rate typically becomes faster. When the atria fibrillate, blood remains in the atria rather than being fully pumped into the ventricle. Blood left in the atria can pool, potentially causing clot formation. The clot is extremely dangerous; it could be pumped out of the heart and circulate throughout the body, possibly becoming lodged in an artery. Typically, the clot will travel to the brain and become lodged there, resulting in a stroke.

- Causes
  - Myocardial infarction
  - CAD
  - High blood pressure (HBP)
  - Pericarditis
  - Myocarditis
  - Pulmonary embolism
  - Pneumonia
  - Hyperthyroidism
  - Obesity
  - Diseases of mitral valves
  - Stimulants (eg, caffeine, nicotine, decongestants, or cocaine)
  - Excessive alcohol consumption
  - Electrocution

- Clinical presentation
  - Chest pain
  - Palpitations
  - Shortness of breath

- o Confusion
- o Dizziness
- o Fainting
- o Fatigue
- o Weakness

□ Management: Atrial fibrillation is managed several ways.

- o Medications (beta-blockers, calcium-channel blockers, or digoxin) for rate control
- o Electrical cardioversion
- o Surgery
- o Pacemaker
- o Anticoagulation, which is required in chronic atrial fibrillation

□ Prevention

- o Low-fat, low-cholesterol diet
- o Regular exercise to maintain a healthy weight
- o Avoid smoking
- o Avoid large amounts of alcohol on a regular basis
- o Diabetics should control blood sugar levels
- o Patients with underlying heart diseases should take medications as prescribed

CORONARY ARTERY DISEASE

□ Also known as: Coronary heart disease (CHD), heart disease, atherosclerosis

□ Description: CAD occurs when plaque (fatty substances) builds up inside the coronary arteries. The coronary arteries are responsible for bringing oxygenated blood to the heart muscle tissue. Increased blockage of these arteries can lead to a heart attack.

- Causes
  - Dyslipidemia
  - Hypertension
  - Diabetes mellitus
  - Obesity
  - Age
  - Family history
  - Sedentary lifestyle
  - High-fat diet
  - Smoking
  - Alcohol abuse
  - Metabolic syndrome such as dyslipidemia, hypertension, central obesity, and impaired glucose tolerance
- Clinical presentation: Some individuals are asymptomatic. Others may experience symptoms when the heart is stressed, such as with exercise.
- Symptoms include the following:
  - Chest pain or discomfort
  - Shortness of breath
  - Heart attack
  - Nausea
  - Increased sweating
  - Racing heartbeat
- Diagnosis: EKG, exercise or thallium stress tests, cardiac catheterization, and coronary angiography
- Management
  - Lifestyle changes including a healthy diet, exercise, and avoiding smoking

- o Medications such as lipid-lowering agents, antihypertensives, and supplements (eg, omega-3 fish oils)

- o Cardiac catheterization in patients with severe disease

DEEP VEIN THROMBOSIS

- □ Also known as: Venous thrombosis, venous thromboembolism (VTE), blood clot

- □ Description: A deep vein thrombosis (DVT) is a blood clot that has formed in a deep vein, normally in the lower extremities or pelvis, but it may occur anywhere in the body. A blood clot that has dislodged and traveled to the lungs is called a pulmonary embolism.

- □ Causes

  - o Poor circulation

  - o Inefficient or abnormal clotting of blood

- □ Risk factors

  - o History of DVT

  - o Prolonged inactivity

  - o Prolonged surgery

  - o Family history

  - o Pregnancy

  - o Cancer

  - o Oral contraceptive use (especially after the age of 35)

  - o Smoking

  - o History of heart failure

  - o Pacemaker

  - o Obesity

- □ Clinical presentation: Often there are no signs and symptoms. DVT may present with the following:

  - o Pain or cramping in the affected extremity

  - o Redness

- o Swelling

- o Increased warmth

- o Positive Homans' sign

- □ Diagnosis: High clinical suspicion. Venous Doppler ultrasound scanning is most commonly used.

- □ Management: Elevation of extremity, compression stockings. Medical treatment with anticoagulants and thrombolytics.

DYSLIPIDEMIA

- □ Description: A condition that contributes to the build-up of plaque in the arteries. It consists of having elevated levels of triglycerides, total plasma cholesterol, and/or low-density lipoprotein (LDL).

- □ Causes

  - o Genetics

  - o Leading a sedentary lifestyle

  - o Eating a high-fat, high-cholesterol diet

  - o Diabetes mellitus

  - o Alcohol abuse

  - o Chronic kidney disease

  - o Hypothyroidism

  - o Primary biliary cirrhosis

  - o Certain medications

- □ Clinical presentation: No presence of signs and symptoms

- □ Management: Initial management is with lifestyle changes such as healthy diet and exercise. Dietary supplements including omega-3 fatty acid fish oil, fiber, and nuts are recommended. Lipid-lowering medications may be required (statins, fibrates, niacin, and resin medications).

HYPERTENSION

- □ Also known as: HBP

- Description: Hypertension is an elevation in blood pressure. Normal reading is 120/80 mm Hg. Prehypertension is 135/85 mm Hg. Hypertension is 140/90 mm Hg. Primary or essential hypertension has no known cause and accounts for 90% to 95% of cases. In 5% to 10% of cases, it is secondary to another condition, such as renal vascular disease; renal parenchymal disease; endocrinologic causes such as pheochromocytoma; Cushing's syndrome; primary hyperaldosteronism; and coarctation of the aorta. Several medications that can elevate blood pressure include oral contraceptives, decongestants, nonsteroidal anti-inflammatories, exogenous thyroid hormone, and appetite suppressants.

- Causes
  - Risk factors include:
    - Family history
    - Obesity
    - Excess dietary salt
    - Smoking
    - Sedentary lifestyle
    - Alcohol abuse
    - Stress
    - Poor overall diet

- Clinical presentation
  - Often no signs or symptoms
  - In cases of extreme elevation, headache and blurred vision can exist
  - Untreated or poorly controlled hypertension can lead to stroke, congestive heart failure, CAD, and renal insufficiency

- Management: Initial management is to make lifestyle changes such as a low-fat, low-sodium diet, incorporate exercise, adequately hydrate, avoid smoking, and limit alcohol intake.

When diet and exercise fail, medications are necessary and commonly include diuretics, angiotensin converting enzyme (ACE) inhibitors, beta-blockers, calcium-channel blockers, and angiotensin-receptor blockers.

HYPOTENSION

- Also known as: Low blood pressure (LBP)

- Description: Hypotension is low blood pressure. A person is considered hypotensive when his or her blood pressure is consistently below 90/60 mm Hg and remains asymptomatic. Hypotension is not considered dangerous or life-threatening unless an individual becomes symptomatic.

- Causes
  - Extended bed rest
  - Trauma with extensive blood loss
  - Serious burns
  - Anaphylaxis
  - Septic shock
  - Pregnancy
  - Cancer
  - Dehydration
  - Medications
  - Adrenal failure
  - Underlying heart issues
  - Underlying endocrine conditions

- Clinical presentation
  - Lightheadedness
  - Dizziness
  - Blurred vision
  - Fatigue
  - Shortness of breath
  - Confusion

- Management: Treatment is warranted if an individual becomes symptomatic. Hypotension can be managed by increasing dietary sodium intake, adequate hydration, and wearing compression stockings. If hypotension is due to an underlying cause, treat the condition.

MYOCARDIAL INFARCTION

- ◻ Also known as: Heart attack
- ◻ Description: A myocardial infarction (MI) is death of heart muscle tissue due to a lack of blood supply.
- ◻ Causes
  - ○ Coronary artery vasospasm
  - ○ Ventricular hypertrophy
  - ○ Coronary artery emboli
  - ○ Cocaine, amphetamines, and ephedrine use
  - ○ Arteritis
  - ○ Other coronary artery abnormalities
- ◻ Risk factors
  - ○ Age
  - ○ Male gender
  - ○ Smoking
  - ○ Dyslipidemia
  - ○ Diabetes mellitus
  - ○ Poorly controlled hypertension
  - ○ Type A personality
  - ○ Family history
  - ○ Sedentary lifestyle
- ◻ Clinical presentation
  - ○ Angina
  - ○ Anxiety

- o Cough

- o Diaphoresis

- o Dyspnea

- o Lightheadedness

- o Nausea

- o Pain in the arms, back, jaw, and neck

- o Syncope

- □ Management: Myocardial infarction is a medical emergency. Treatment includes oxygen therapy, aspirin, and nitroglycerin. Beta blockers, heparin, and morphine are also given. Further therapeutic interventions include administration of fibrinolytics, angiography with stent placement, and coronary artery bypass surgery.

- □ Prevention

- o Maintain a healthy, low-fat diet

- o Maintain a healthy weight

- o No smoking

- o Regular exercise

- o Maintain low cholesterol, low blood pressure, and control blood sugar.

PALPITATIONS

- □ Description: Palpitations are heart beats that feel abnormally rapid or unusual. Patients commonly refer to palpitations by saying, "My heart felt like it was beating out of my chest."

- □ Causes

- o Exercise

- o Anxiety

- o Fever

- o Stimulants (eg, caffeine, nicotine, diet pills, cocaine)

- o Overactive thyroid

- o Anemia
- o Hyperventilation
- o Mitral valve prolapse
- o Heart disease
- o Medications
- □ Clinical presentation
  - o Varying heart beat speeds and feelings (eg, rapid, racing, fluttering, irregular)
  - o Contact 911 if the following symptoms accompany palpitations:
    - Angina
    - Dizziness
    - Syncope
- □ Management: Treat the underlying cause.
- □ Prevention
  - o Stress management
  - o Maintain a healthy, low-fat diet
  - o Maintain good cholesterol, blood pressure, and blood sugar levels
  - o Avoid smoking
  - o Exercise

PERIPHERAL ARTERIAL DISEASE

- □ Also known as: Peripheral artery disease (PAD), atherosclerotic peripheral arterial disease, peripheral vascular disease (PVD), vascular disease, or hardening of the arteries.
- □ Description: A circulatory disease with narrowing of blood vessels due to plaque build-up. Narrowing of the blood vessels leads to reduced blood flow through the affected arteries.

- Causes
  - Atherosclerosis (main cause)
  - Blood clots
  - Infection
- Risk factors
  - High cholesterol
  - Obesity
  - Smoking
  - Age
  - Diabetes mellitus
  - Family history
  - Hypertension
- Clinical presentation
  - Cramping in the extremities, especially the calf muscles
  - A feeling of coldness in the extremities
  - Numbness in the extremities
  - Reduced hair growth on the extremities
  - Skin discoloration
  - Poor toe- or fingernail growth
- Management
  - Exercise
  - Maintain a low-fat, healthy diet
  - Maintain good levels of cholesterol, blood pressure, and blood sugar
  - Avoid smoking
  - Take medications as prescribed

- o Medical procedures

  - Angioplasty

  - Bypass surgery

  - Thrombolytic therapy

- □ Diagnostic testing

  - o Physical exam

  - o Ankle brachial-index (ABI)

  - o Ultrasound

  - o Angiography

  - o Blood test

- □ Additional information: If not taken care of, PAD can result in gangrene, stroke, or heart attack.

SHOCK

- □ Description: A decrease in adequate perfusion of oxygenated blood throughout the body. Shock is a life-threatening emergency.

- □ Causes: There are several different types of shock, characterized by cause. Most common causes include the following:

  - o Hypovolemic shock—Shock resulting from low circulating blood volume

  - o Hemorrhagic shock—Shock resulting from severe hemorrhage

  - o Neurogenic shock—Shock resulting from impairment of the nerve conduction, resulting in the inability to control blood vessel diameter, causing systemic vasodilation.

  - o Cardiogenic shock—Shock resulting from impaired cardiac output as in a myocardial infarction

  - o Anaphylactic shock—Shock resulting from a systemic allergic reaction to a toxin in the body

  - o Septic shock—Shock resulting from a massive systemic infection

- Clinical presentation
  - Anxiety
  - Cool, clammy skin (septic shock may exhibit warm, moist skin)
  - Diaphoresis
  - Fatigue
  - Hypotension
  - Pale skin/loss of normal skin complexion
  - Priapism (in neurogenic shock)
  - Rapid, shallow breathing
  - Thirst
  - Weak, rapid pulse
- Anaphylactic shock exhibits different symptoms, including:
  - Difficulty breathing
  - Narrowing of the airway due to swelling
  - Swelling of the face
  - Urticaria
  - Warm, flushed skin
- Management: Shock is a medical emergency and will likely require aggressive intravenous therapy (normal saline bolus) to increase volume. When treating victims of trauma, preventative measures should be implemented. These include laying the victim on a flat surface, elevating the legs 8 to 12 inches, and maintaining normal body temperature. In cases of anaphylactic shock, administration of epinephrine is essential as a life-saving intervention.
- Other important information: It is important to note that health care providers may be able to prevent or minimize shock in the out-of-hospital setting. However, shock cannot be reversed in the field without advanced care.

SUPRAVENTRICULAR TACHYCARDIA

- Also known as: Paroxysmal supraventricular tachycardia (PSVT), paroxysmal atrial tachycardia (PAT)

- Description: Tachycardia is a condition in which the heart beats in excess of 100 beats per minute. SVT happens when the tachycardia originates above the ventricles. PSVT is a tachycardic rhythm that involves an accessory pathway in the electrical conduction system of the heart.

- Causes
  - Hyperthyroidism
  - Stimulants (eg, caffeine, diet pills, cocaine)
  - Alcohol abuse
  - Certain medications
  - Chronic obstructive pulmonary disease (COPD)
  - Pneumonia
  - Illegal drug use

- Clinical presentation
  - Angina
  - Dizziness
  - Labored breathing
  - Lightheadedness
  - Loss of consciousness
  - Palpitations

- Management
  - Medications (eg, beta-blockers, calcium-channel blockers, antiarrhythmic agents)
  - Vagal maneuvers, such as coughing or gagging
  - Electrical cardioversion
  - Catheter ablation

- ❑ Other important information
    - o Diagnosis is made through EKG interpretation.
- ❑ Prevention
    - o Limit alcohol
    - o No smoking
    - o Limit caffeine
    - o Stress management
    - o Avoid over-the-counter decongestants

VENTRICULAR FIBRILLATION

- ❑ Also known as: V-fib
- ❑ Description: A condition in which the ventricles of the heart beat irregularly and rapidly and do not produce a coordinated contraction. Ventricular fibrillation is a potentially fatal cardiac arrhythmia. Patients experiencing ventricular fibrillation are considered to be in cardiac arrest.
- ❑ Clinical presentation
    - o Unresponsiveness
    - o Lack of carotid pulse
    - o Respiratory arrest
- ❑ Management
    - o Cardiopulmonary resuscitation
    - o Defibrillation
    - o Advanced cardiac life support (ACLS)

VENTRICULAR TACHYCARDIA

- ❑ Also known as: V-tach
- ❑ Description: Three or more ectopic ventricular complexes with a heart rate of over 100 beats per minute. Sustained ventricular tachycardia for greater than 30 seconds can lead to cardiac arrest.

- Causes
    - Previous heart disease
    - Electrolyte imbalances
    - Medications
    - Over-the-counter decongestants
    - Illegal drugs
- Clinical presentation
    - Chest pain or discomfort
    - Dyspnea
    - Palpitations
    - Syncope
- Management
    - Advanced cardiac life support protocols
    - Defibrillation
    - Implantable cardioverter defibrillator (ICD)
    - Antiarrhythmic medications
- Other important information: Diagnosis is confirmed through EKG interpretation

2

PULMONARY CONDITIONS

- ☐ Asthma
- ☐ Acute bronchitis
- ☐ Chronic obstructive pulmonary disease
- ☐ Cystic fibrosis
- ☐ Pneumonia
- ☐ Pulmonary embolism
- ☐ Influenza
- ☐ Pulmonary tuberculosis

Rehberg RS, Rehberg JS.
Cram Session in General Medical Conditions:
A Handbook for Students & Clinicians (pp. 19-30).
© 2012 Taylor & Francis Group.

ASTHMA

- □ Description: Chronic, reversible airway obstruction. Allergies and inhaled environmental allergens cause inflammation which leads to increased airway secretions and bronchospasm, resulting in constriction. Symptoms reverse spontaneously or with the inhalation of medications.

- □ Triggering factors
  - o Smoke
  - o Pollutants
  - o Viral infection
  - o Temperature change
  - o Cold air
  - o Exercise

- □ Clinical presentation
  - o Wheezing
  - o Cough
  - o Chest tightness
  - o Shortness of breath
  - o With increasing severity of the attack:
    - ▪ Retractions
    - ▪ Tachycardia
    - ▪ Fatigue
    - ▪ Cyanosis

- □ Management: The goal of treatment is to alleviate symptoms, reduce inflammation, and prevent exacerbations by recognizing triggering factors. Medications include inhaled short-acting beta$_2$-agonists, inhaled corticosteroids, long-acting beta$_2$-agonists, systemic corticosteroids, inhaled cromolyn, inhaled nedocromil, leukotriene modifiers, methylxanthines, and immunomodulators. Treatment regimens vary depending on the frequency and severity of attacks. Severe asthma (status asthmaticus) is a medical emergency.

ACUTE BRONCHITIS

☐ Description: Inflammation of the upper respiratory tract, specifically the trachea and bronchi. The infectious agent is typically viral; also caused by *Mycoplasma pneumoniae* and *Chlamydia pneumonia.*

☐ Clinical presentation

o Fever

o Cough

o Wheezing

o Sputum production

o Cough may last 3 to 4 weeks

☐ Management: Routine use of antibiotics is not indicated. Analgesics and antipyretics should be used as needed. Bronchodilators may be of some use. Antitussives can be used in cough persisting for longer than 2 weeks.

CHRONIC OBSTRUCTIVE PULMONARY DISEASE

☐ Also known as: COPD

☐ Description: Chronic obstructive pulmonary disease (COPD) is a respiratory condition characterized by chronic dyspnea due to the presence of expiratory airflow obstruction resulting from chronic bronchitis, emphysema, or both. The condition is generally progressive. With emphysema, there is permanent distension of the air spaces distal to the terminal bronchioles with destruction of the alveolar walls.

☐ Clinical presentation

o Chronic bronchitis—Patient is termed *blue bloater*

■ Excessive mucous secretions and productive cough for at least 3 months for 2 consecutive years

■ Rhonchi are present upon chest exam; wheezing is common

■ Individual appears cyanotic and may be edematous

■ Patients are typically overweight

- o Emphysema—Patient is termed *pink puffer*

  - ▪ Shortness of breath

  - ▪ Breath sounds are quiet on chest exam

  - ▪ Breathing is uncomfortable

  - ▪ Individuals are commonly thin

- □ Chest x-ray and pulmonary function testing are useful in establishing diagnosis.

- □ Management: Management is to minimize risk factors. Smoking cessation is encouraged. Oxygen therapy is useful. Pharmacotherapy use depends on the severity of the disease and includes short-acting bronchodilators, long-acting bronchodilators, long-acting anticholinergics, inhaled corticosteroids, oral corticosteroids, or any combinations of these.

- □ Additional information: Administrations of influenza and pneumococcal vaccines are recommended.

CYSTIC FIBROSIS

- □ Description: Cystic fibrosis (CF) is the most common lethal inherited disease of the White population. It is an autosomal-recessive disorder. A genetic mutation leaves cells impermeable to chloride, making salt-rich secretions. Sweat becomes salty. Thick, viscous mucous is produced throughout the body, obstructing glands and ducts. The average lifespan for those with the disease is 35 years. Pulmonary manifestations cause the most morbidity and mortality. Chronic inflammation and infections with acute exacerbations lead to respiratory failure. Other manifestations are gastrointestinal, genitourinary, and skeletal (including meconium ileus), pancreatic insufficiency, malnutrition, failure to thrive, diabetes mellitus, biliary cirrhosis, cholelithiasis, male infertility, and growth retardation.

- □ Diagnostic testing

  - o Sweat test—The gold standard for diagnosing CF

  - o Chest x-ray

- o Pulmonary function tests
- o Sputum cultures
- ☐ Clinical presentation
  - o Pulmonary
    - Progressive cough
    - Purulent sputum
    - Dyspnea
    - Hemoptysis
    - Wheezing
    - Rales
    - Digital clubbing
    - Nasal polyps
  - o Gastrointestinal
    - Abdominal distension
    - Greasy stools
    - Feeding intolerance
    - Increased flatulence
- ☐ Management
  - o For pulmonary disease
    - Antibiotics; chest physiotherapy; bronchodilators; anti-inflammatories, both steroidal and nonsteroidal; mucolytics; and oxygen therapy. Lung transplantation is considered with severe disease.
  - o For gastrointestinal disease
    - Pancreatic enzyme supplementation and caloric supplements are used. Patients should be referred for nutritional advice.

PNEUMONIA

- ☐ Description: Lower respiratory tract infection that is classified as community-acquired or hospital-acquired.

    - o Community-acquired pneumonia (CAP): Occurs outside of the hospital

    - o Hospital-acquired pneumonia (HAP)/Nosocomial: Occurs more than 48 hours after admission to health care facility

With CAP, the pathogen is usually bacterial, most commonly *Streptococcus pneumoniae. Mycoplasma pneumoniae, Haemophilus influenzae, Chlamydia pneumoniae*, and respiratory viruses are less common.

With HAP, the pathogens are commonly *Pseudomonas aeruginosa, Staphylococcus aureus, Klebsiella pneumoniae, Escherichia coli*, and *enterobacter.*

- ☐ Clinical presentation

    - o Fever

    - o Dyspnea

    - o Cough, either productive or nonproductive

    - o Headache

    - o Fatigue

    - o Myalgias

    - o Chest discomfort

    - o Tachypnea, rales, or crackles

- ☐ Chest x-ray is used to help confirm diagnosis.

- ☐ Management: Treatment is empirical as it can be difficult to differentiate the cause. In HAP, treatment depends on the severity of the disease and the length of hospitalization. Oral antimicrobials such as macrolides, doxycycline, fluoroquinolones, and beta-lactams are used. Adequate hydration, oxygen therapy, antipyretics, and analgesics are used as needed.

- ☐ Additional information: Immunization is available for those over the age of 65 and for those under 2 years of age with comorbidities.

PULMONARY EMBOLISM

- Description: Blood flow to the lungs is obstructed by venous thrombus, usually from deep vein thrombosis (DVT), but upper extremity thrombosis and catheter-associated thrombosis can also cause pulmonary embolism (PE). PE can result in sudden death.

- Risk factors
  - Periods of immobility
  - Recent prolonged surgery
  - Estrogen therapy
  - Pregnancy
  - Smoking
  - Stroke
  - Cancer
  - Leg fractures
  - Previous DVT/PE
  - Genetic or acquired thrombophilia

- Diagnostic testing
  - Electrocardiogram (EKG)
  - Arterial blood gas
  - Chest x-ray
  - Ventilation-perfusion scans (V/Q scan)
  - Enzyme-linked immunosorbent assay (ELISA) D-Dimer test
  - Computed tomography (CT) scan of the chest
  - Pulmonary angiography

- Clinical presentation
  - Sudden onset of breathlessness
  - Chest pain
  - Dyspnea

- o Hemoptysis

- o Syncope

- o Palpitations

- o Tachycardia

- o Hypotension

- o Tachypnea

- o Loud P_2 (pulmonic component of second heart sound)

- o Increased jugular venous pressure (JVP)

- o Right ventricular rub and gallop

- o Look for signs of lower extremity DVT

- □ Management: Supportive care including oxygen therapy and intravenous (IV) saline infusion.

- □ IV heparin (anticoagulant) should be started when there is a high clinical suspicion of PE, even before confirmatory testing, as long as no contraindication exists. Thrombolytic therapy (streptokinase, urokinase, or tissue plasminogen activator [TPA]) will help destroy a clot. Pulmonary embolectomy is rarely performed. Oral anticoagulants are begun once the individual is stable and are continued for at least 3 months. Inferior vena cava (IVC) filter placement is used to prevent recurrent emboli.

INFLUENZA

- □ Also known as: Flu

- □ Description: Influenza viruses are an orthomyxovirus of 3 types: A, B, and C. Influenza A causes severe outbreaks. Influenza B outbreaks are less severe. An influenza C infection typically results in mild respiratory illness, or may produce no symptoms at all. Outbreaks typically occur in the late fall and winter months.

- □ Diagnosis: Usually clinically made. Rapid influenza tests using nasopharyngeal swabbings are available for aiding the diagnosis.

□ Clinical presentation

    o Abrupt onset of fever

    o Chills

    o Headache

    o Coryza

    o Pharyngitis

    o Cough

    o Myalgias

    o Malaise

□ Management: Supportive care. Oseltamivir and zanamivir are antiviral medications used for both the treatment and prophylaxis of influenza. For treatment, medications must be given within 48 hours of the onset of symptoms.

□ Additional information: Influenza infection can be minimized or prevented through frequent hand washing, covering the mouth when coughing and/or sneezing, and annual vaccination.

PULMONARY TUBERCULOSIS

□ Also known as: TB

□ Description: Systemic disease caused by the mycobacterium tuberculosis (TB), frequently presenting as pulmonary tuberculosis. Infection is transmitted via the respiratory route. Of those individuals exposed, only 30% develop infection. Of those infected, only 10% develop primary TB; the remainder develop latent TB infection. Typically, active TB is the result of reactivation of infection in those with LTBI, not primary infection. Other systemic manifestations of tuberculosis infection are termed *extrapulmonary*.

- ☐ Diagnostic testing
  - ○ Latent infection
    - Tuberculin skin testing (TST)
    - Mantoux test (most commonly used)—purified protein derivative (PPD) is injected intradermally.
    - Diameter of induration is measured 48 to 72 hours later.
    - Specific criterion exists for interpretation of the Mantoux test.
  - ○ Active infection
    - Sputum culture
    - Fluorochrome staining and acid-fast staining of sputum can be used for screening
    - Bronchoscopy for biopsy can be performed
    - Chest x-ray
      - Infiltrates are located in the apical, posterior upper lobe
      - In elderly patients, infiltrate with pleural effusion can be seen in the lower lobe
- ☐ Clinical presentation
  - ○ Primary TB is often asymptomatic
  - ○ Active TB
    - Fatigue
    - Malaise
    - Low-grade fever
    - Night sweats
    - Chronic cough

- Weight loss

- Anorexia

- If extrapulmonary systems are involved, symptoms are related to the involved organ system

☐ Management: Initial therapy of pulmonary TB includes the use of 4 medications. Dosage schedules and regimens vary:

o Isoniazid (INH)

o Rifampin (RIF)

o Pyrazinamide (PZA)

o Ethambutol (EMB)

☐ To reduce the risk of conversion to active disease, chemoprophylaxis should be administered to the following:

o Individuals < 35 years of age with a positive skin testing (+PPD)

o Individuals with immunosuppression or HIV-infection who have been exposed to or have a +PPD

o Those in close contact with patients who have newly diagnosed active TB

o Individuals with a history of untreated TB or positive chest x-ray (without active disease)

o Individuals with +PPD and risk factors for developing active disease

o Individuals known to have converted a +PPD within 1 year

3

NEUROLOGICAL CONDITIONS

- ☐ Alzheimer's disease
- ☐ Amyotrophic lateral sclerosis
- ☐ Bell's palsy
- ☐ Cerebral vascular accident
- ☐ Dementia
- ☐ Epilepsy
- ☐ Guillain-Barré syndrome
- ☐ Headaches
- ☐ Multiple sclerosis
- ☐ Myasthenia gravis
- ☐ Parkinson's disease
- ☐ Tourette syndrome

Rehberg RS, Rehberg JS.
*Cram Session in General Medical Conditions:
A Handbook for Students & Clinicians* (pp. 31-48).
© 2012 Taylor & Francis Group.

ALZHEIMER'S DISEASE

□ Also known as: Dementia, senile dementia

□ Description: An incurable, degenerative form of dementia. Alzheimer's is the most common form of dementia, and is most commonly diagnosed in people over the age of 65.

□ Causes: Researchers believe that Alzheimer's disease is caused by a build-up of proteins in the brain, which result in the formation of plaque, or deposits of protein that accumulate in spaces between nerve cells, and tangles, which are deposits of protein that accumulate inside nerve cells.

□ Clinical presentation: The most common and early symptom of Alzheimer's is difficulty remembering recently learned information. Other symptoms may include the following:

  o Acquired difficulties in speaking and/or writing

  o Challenges in problem solving

  o Confusion

  o Difficulty interpreting visual images or spatial relationships

  o Difficulty completing routine tasks

  o Impaired or poor judgment

  o Inability to retrace steps

  o Mood and personality changes

  o Social withdrawal

□ Management: There is no cure for Alzheimer's disease. However, treatment options and medications that address cognitive and behavioral symptoms do exist.

AMYOTROPHIC LATERAL SCLEROSIS

□ Also known as: Lou Gehrig's disease

□ Description: Amyotrophic lateral sclerosis (ALS) is a progressive neurodegenerative disease that is usually fatal. ALS attacks the neurons in the brain and spinal cord, leading to muscle atrophy. The disorder is characterized by muscle weakness and atrophy throughout the body as a result of the degeneration of both the upper and lower motor neurons. Paralysis affects patients in later stages. Respiratory difficulty is caused when muscles in the chest area begin to atrophy.

- Causes: The definitive cause of ALS is still unknown. Genetic defect is a factor in approximately 20% of cases.

- Clinical presentation
  - Respiratory distress
  - Difficulty swallowing
    - Gagging
    - Chokes easily
  - Head drop due to weakened spinal and neck muscles
  - Muscle cramping
  - Progressive muscle weakness/atrophy
    - Commonly involves one part of the body first, such as the arm or hand
    - Eventually leads to difficulty lifting, climbing stairs, and walking
  - Paralysis
  - Speech problems, such as a slow or abnormal speech pattern
  - Voice changes, hoarseness

- Additional symptoms that may be associated with this disease:
  - Drooling
  - Muscle contractions
  - Muscle spasms
  - Ankle, foot, and leg swelling
  - Weight loss

- Management: There is no known cure for ALS. Pharmacotherapy, along with physical therapy, rehabilitation, use of braces, a wheelchair, or other orthopedic measures may be indicated to maximize muscle function and general health. Some patients may need to have a feeding tube placed in their stomach since choking is a common symptom. The use of assistive ventilatory devices, such as a continuous positive airway pressure (CPAP) device, is a common treatment and is only used during sleep.

BELL'S PALSY

☐ Description: Sudden, temporary form of unilateral facial paralysis or weakness resulting from damage to the facial nerve (cranial nerve VII), which controls movement of the muscles in the face and mouth. In some cases, this condition can affect sense of taste as well as tear and saliva production.

☐ Causes: In most cases, Bell's palsy is caused by a reactivation of the herpes virus. Other viral and bacterial infections may also cause the condition.

☐ Clinical presentation

  o Change in facial expression (grimacing)

  o Difficulty eating and drinking

  o Drooling due to lack of control over facial muscles

  o Droopy eyelid or corner of the mouth

  o Dry eye or mouth

  o The face feels stiff or pulled to one side

  o Facial paralysis of one side of the face, making it hard to close 1 eye

  o Headache

  o Loss of sense of taste

  o Pain behind or in front of the ear

  o Sensitivity to sound (hyperacusis) on the affected side of the face

  o Twitching or weakness in the face

☐ Management: Most cases recover within 1 to 2 months. The primary treatment goal is relief of symptoms. Corticosteroids and/or antiviral medication may be prescribed.

CEREBROVASCULAR ACCIDENT

- Also known as: Stroke, brain attack

- Description: A stroke occurs when there is a disruption of oxygenated blood supply to the brain. Ischemic stroke, the most common form, occurs when an artery carrying blood to the brain is blocked. Causes of blockage include narrowing of the arteries due to atherosclerosis or a blood clot (thrombus or embolus). Hemorrhagic stroke occurs when an artery carrying blood to the brain ruptures, either due to traumatic injury or as a result of an aneurysm that has ruptured. Interruption of blood flow causes brain cell damage due to the lack of oxygen. Resulting symptoms of a stroke can be temporary or permanent and range from mild to severe.

- Clinical presentation

  o Changes in level of consciousness

  o Unilateral facial drooping

  o Sudden numbness, decrease, or loss of function of the face, arm, or leg, usually affecting one side of the body

  o Sudden severe headache

  o Vision disturbances

  o Unequal pupils

  o Vertigo

  o Loss of balance or coordination

  o Sensory disturbances (hearing, taste, smell, vision, touch)

  o Mental confusion

  o Difficulty speaking or swallowing

  o Loss of bowel and/or bladder control

- Management: Health care providers should offer immediate care to the stroke patient by protecting the airway, assessing vital signs, performing a detailed history and physical exam, and administering high flow oxygen, if trained. Early recognition and treatment usually improves patient outcome, especially in ischemic stroke. Stroke assessment scales, such as the Cincinnati Stroke Scale, can be useful in detecting stroke. The patient who has abnormal findings on any one of these 3 exam points may be experiencing an acute stroke:

o Facial Droop

- Normal: Both sides of face move equally well.

- Abnormal: One side of face does not move, or does not move as well as other side.

o Arm Drift

- Normal: Both arms move the same, or both arms don't move at all.

- Abnormal: One arm doesn't move or one arm drifts down compared to the other.

o Speech: Ask the patient to repeat the following phrase: "You can't teach an old dog new tricks."

- Normal: Patient says correct words without slurring speech.

- Abnormal: Patient slurs words, says wrong words, or is unable to speak.

Patients exhibiting signs and symptoms of stroke should be transported to the nearest hospital immediately. Recent advances in the treatment of ischemic stroke can often provide the patient with a favorable prognosis if treatment is initiated immediately.

Treatment for ischemic stroke normally involves thrombolytic therapy, which dissolves clots and restores blood flow. Blood thinners may also be prescribed. For hemorrhagic strokes, surgery is often required to remove blood and repair the damaged vessels. For long term treatment, one must go through occupational, physical, and speech therapy to try to recover as much function as possible and to prevent future strokes. Elderly patients who suffer through strokes often have a harder recovery; thus, the majority end up in rehabilitation centers and nursing homes.

□ Additional information: Controllable risk factors for stroke include hypertension, high cholesterol, smoking, diabetes, artery disease, poor diet, physical inactivity, obesity, sickle cell disease, and heart disease. Risk factors for stroke that cannot be controlled include age, heredity, race, gender, and previous history of stroke.

Transient ischemic attacks (TIAs or "mini" strokes) are considered warning strokes that produce stroke-like symptoms but do not pose lasting effects. Individuals who experience TIAs are at greater risk for stroke and should be evaluated by a physician.

DEMENTIA

☐ Description: A loss of brain function, usually irreversible, that occurs with certain diseases. It affects memory, thinking, language, judgment, and behavior.

☐ Causes: Dementia usually occurs in older patients. Various medical conditions can lead to dementia, including the following:

- A small stroke

- Lyme disease

- Human immunodeficiency virus (HIV) or acquired immunodeficiency syndrome (AIDS)

- Parkinson's disease

- Huntington's disease

- Pick's disease

- Multiple sclerosis

☐ Clinical presentation: Dementia affects a person's brain functioning. Most often the first sign is short-term memory loss. Symptoms of dementia are often categorized by stages: early, intermediate, and late.

- Early stages of dementia

  - Difficulty remembering—Learning and retaining new information becomes extremely difficult

  - Difficulty with otherwise simple tasks such as word recognition, elementary math, remembering where they put items, or finding their way to places they have been many times before

  - Personality changes

  - Social isolation

- o Intermediate stages
  - Inability to learn or retain new information
  - Assistance is needed with basic daily activities like eating and bathing
  - Personality changes progress, leading to behavioral issues
  - Loss of sense of time and place
  - Confusion, even in familiar areas
  - Depression leading to altered sensation, hallucinations, and paranoia
- o End stages
  - Inability to perform fundamental daily activities
  - Difficulty understanding language
  - Difficulty recognizing family members
  - Inability to swallow, putting the individual at risk of malnutrition
- ☐ Management: Patient safety is the number 1 goal in the treatment of dementia. The living environment must be examined to assist in the prevention of accidents. Medication may be used to treat the patient's behavioral disorders. The patient should be medically evaluated regularly to address conditions that increase the patient's chances of mental confusion (eg, vision or hearing loss, depression, and nutritional deficiencies).

EPILEPSY

- ☐ Also known as: Seizure disorder
- ☐ Description: A neurological condition usually diagnosed after 2 or more seizures that were not caused by trauma, hypoglycemia, or alcohol withdrawal. Unusual excited electrical activity in the brain produces abnormal movements and/or behavior.
- ☐ Causes
  - o Unknown
  - o Heredity

o Brain injury

o Brain tumor

o Stroke

o Infection

o Atherosclerosis

o Degenerative conditions such as Alzheimer's disease

☐ Clinical presentation: Seizures are classified as focal (also known as partial) seizures or generalized seizures, which include a wide range of symptoms ranging from full-body stiffening and convulsions to absence seizures characterized a blank stare. Some patients may experience an aura or unusual sensations (such as headaches and sensory abnormalities) preceding an actual seizure.

o Focal seizures

■ Emotional or behavioral changes

■ Repetitious movements (automatisms) such as blinking or twitching

■ Patient experiences unusual taste, smell, feel, or sound

■ Jerking movement of one part of the body

■ Vertigo

■ Tingling

■ Vision disturbances

o Generalized seizures

■ A staring spell or subtle body movements which may cause loss of consciousness (absence seizures)

■ Sudden jerks or twitches of a patient's arms and legs (myoclonic seizures)

■ Sudden loss of muscle tone, causing patient to collapse (atonic seizures)

■ Loss of consciousness, uncontrollable body stiffening and/or jerking, and possible loss of bowel and/or bladder control (tonic-clonic or grand mal)

❑ Management: Acute management of any seizure includes protecting the patient from injury. Do not attempt to restrain the patient during a seizure. Instead, move away objects that could cause injury if struck by the patient during a convulsive episode. Place a blanket, jacket, or other form of padding behind the head. Do not attempt to place objects in the mouth. Emergency medical services should be activated in cases where the cause of the seizure is due to fever, head trauma, or alcohol/drug use; if the victim's medical history is unknown; if a victim has never had a seizure; or when a seizure lasts more than 5 minutes in a patient who has a positive diagnosis/history of epilepsy.

Antiepileptic drugs are often used to reduce the number of seizures. Patients taking antiepileptic medications may experience side effects such as sedation, fatigue, vertigo, and weight gain. Surgery may be indicated in patients experiencing seizures as a result of a tumor, abnormal bleeding in vessels, or other brain abnormalities. A ketogenic diet, (high fat, low carbohydrate) may decrease the frequency of seizures and is often used in treating children with the condition.

GUILLAIN-BARRÉ SYNDROME

❑ Description: A rare but severe autoimmune condition that attacks the peripheral nervous system, causing weakness and numbness in the extremities and can lead to loss of deep tendon reflexes and paralysis of the entire body.

❑ Causes: The cause of Guillain-Barré syndrome is not completely understood. However, the condition most often presents in the days or weeks following respiratory or gastrointestinal viral infection. Surgery and vaccination have also been known to trigger this condition. The onset of Guillain-Barré can be rapid (hours, days) or slow (3 to 4 weeks).

❑ Clinical presentation

o Initial symptoms

■ Weakness and/or tingling sensation in the lower extremity, eventually spreading to the upper extremity

■ Difficulty breathing

■ Difficulty controlling eye and facial movement

■ Difficulty speaking, chewing, and swallowing

Symptoms may eventually intensify, leading to complete paralysis. Paralysis may lead to respiratory arrest and require artificial respiration. The inability of the patient to regulate heart rate and blood pressure is a common complication.

□ Management: There is no known cure for Guillain-Barré syndrome, but therapies can lessen the severity of the illness and accelerate recovery in most patients. Plasmapheresis and high-dose immunoglobulin therapy are used to treat the syndrome. Plasmapheresis seems to reduce the severity and duration of the Guillain-Barré episode. The most critical part of the treatment for this syndrome consists of keeping the patient's body functioning during recovery of the nervous system. This can sometimes require placing the patient on a respirator, a heart monitor, or other machines that assist body function. Although life threatening, most patients recover from this condition, even in severe cases. Some patients will experience a lasting degree of muscle weakness.

HEADACHES (INCLUDING MIGRAINE, CLUSTER, AND TENSION)

□ Also known as: Cephalgia

□ Description: Pain that occurs in the head and upper neck. It is considered one of the most common locations of pain in the body. Headaches are classified as either primary or secondary headaches. Primary headaches are not associated with other pathology.

  o Migraine (disabling pain lasting several hours or days)—Occurs in women more often than men; a family history may exist. It is believed to be the result of abnormal brainstem activity that leads to rapid vasoconstriction of blood vessels in the brain; the triggers may include specific foods or medications, changes in sleep patterns, changes in environmental conditions, stress, fatigue, visual stimulus (such as bright lights), or odors.

  o Cluster—Sudden, with severe pain behind one of the eyes. They occur in bunches or "clusters" for days or months. The cause of cluster headache is also poorly understood. Several theories exist, including vascular abnormalities, trigeminal nerve pathology, and/or abnormal chemical changes in the head.

  o Tension—Occurs most frequently and is the result of contraction of the muscles that cover the skull; tension headaches often occur in individuals experiencing physical or emotional stress.

Secondary headaches are caused by associated diseases including brain tumor, stroke, meningitis, subarachnoid hemorrhage, caffeine withdrawal, or the discontinuation of analgesic medication.

- Triggering factors
  - Migraine
    - Stress
    - Certain foods (alcohol, cheese, chocolate, or monosodium glutamate [MSG])
    - Environmental factors
    - Use of birth control pills
  - Cluster
    - Stress
    - Temperature or barometric pressure changes
    - Seasonal allergies
    - Foods
    - Use of tobacco products
  - Tension
    - Physical and/or emotional stress
- Clinical Presentation
  - A general feeling of discomfort
  - Confusion
  - Hearing impairment
  - Irritability
  - Malaise
  - Nausea
  - Pain in head
  - Visual impairment (blurred vision)
  - Vomiting

□ Management: Management of headaches varies by type. Rest, massage, or heat applied to the back of the upper neck can be effective in relieving tension headaches. Drugs such as acetaminophen, aspirin, and ibuprofen are used for tension headaches. Migraine headaches may respond to nonsteroidal anti-inflammatory drugs (NSAIDs), or migraine-specific medications that contain a combination of drugs. Cluster headaches are often treated with high-flow oxygen, abortive medication, and steroids. Surgery and alternative treatments are other options for the management of cluster headaches. Preventative therapy is an important management option for patients with cluster headaches.

MULTIPLE SCLEROSIS

□ Also known as: MS

□ Description: An autoimmune disease in which the body's immune system attacks the myelin sheath that covers the nerves of the brain and spinal cord, resulting in interference or disruption of nerve impulses between the brain and body. Ultimately, this may result in irreversible deterioration of the nerves. Multiple sclerosis (MS) affects more women than men and often begins between the ages of 20 and 45.

□ Causes: The cause of MS is unknown. It is suspected, however, that viral, environmental, and genetic factors may be potential causes.

□ Clinical presentation: Patients with MS may experience one or more of the following:

  o Vision problems

  o Eye pain

  o Muscle weakness

  o Muscle spasticity

  o Difficulty with gait, balance, and coordination

  o Depression

  o Memory problems

  o Dizziness and vertigo

  o Paresthesia

- o Pain

- o Emotional changes

- o Fatigue

- o Sexual dysfunction

- o Bowel and/or bladder dysfunction

- o Deterioration of cognitive function

- Management: There is no cure for MS. However, there are effective strategies that are available that can slow or minimize exacerbations of the disease. Long-term therapeutic medications that target the immune system can decrease the frequency and duration of exacerbations of the disease. Steroids are also used to decrease the severity of symptoms during an exacerbation. Physical, occupational, and speech therapy may be necessary. A healthy, active lifestyle and proper diet can help slow the progression of the disease. Patients who experience more progressive or advanced symptoms may require the use of assistive devices such as wheelchairs or walkers.

MYASTHENIA GRAVIS

- Description: A chronic autoimmune neuromuscular disorder characterized as weakness of the voluntary muscles of the body. Muscle weakness increases with activity and improves with rest. Muscles that control facial and eyelid movements, chewing, swallowing, and talking are often involved. In more severe cases, muscles that control breathing, the neck, and extremity movement are also involved.

- Causes: This condition is caused by a defect in the transmission of nerve impulses at the neuromuscular junction, which prevents contraction of the voluntary muscles. In healthy nerve conduction, acetylcholine is released when impulses travel through nerves. The acetylcholine binds to receptors that activate muscle contraction. In patients with myasthenia gravis, antibodies block, alter, or even destroy the receptors and muscle contraction is hindered. Pathology of the thymus gland is also thought to be a possible cause of myasthenia gravis.

- Clinical presentation

  - o Muscle weakness, including the following:

    - ▪ Difficulty chewing

    - ▪ Difficulty climbing stairs

- Difficulty lifting objects

- Difficulty talking

- Drooping head

- Muscles that function best after rest

- Need to use hands to rise from a sitting position

- Paralysis

- Difficulty swallowing, frequent gagging, or choking

o Vision problems

- Difficulty maintaining steady gaze

- Double vision

- Eyelid drooping

o Additional symptoms that may be associated with this disease are as follows:

- Breathing difficulty

- Drooling

- Facial paralysis

- Fatigue

- Hoarseness or changing voice

□ Management: Myasthenia gravis can be controlled using medications that improve neuromuscular transmission and increase muscle strength. Immunosuppressive drugs are also used to improve muscular strength by suppressing production of the abnormal antibodies. Intravenous immunoglobulin—which temporarily modifies the immune system and provides the body with normal antibodies from donated blood—is sometimes used when other pharmacotherapy fails. Surgical removal of the thymus is another treatment option.

PARKINSON'S DISEASE

□ Also known as: PD

□ Description: A motor system disorder in which there is a decrease in dopamine-producing cells in the brain. Dopamine, a neurotransmitter, plays a critical role in nerve transmission between the substantia nigra and the corpus striatum, which is required for smooth coordinated muscle movement. The decrease in dopamine results in abnormal nerve firing patterns, which results in impaired movements. This condition progresses slowly over time.

- Causes: A definitive cause is unknown.

- Clinical presentation

  o Tremors of the hands, arms, legs, face, or jaw

  o Impaired balance and coordination

  o Postural instability

  o Rigidity or stiffness of the trunk

  o Slow movement

- Management: There is no cure for this disease. However, there are various therapies and medications that can provide relief. Each patient's treatment plan is unique depending on age, work status, family, and living situation. Medications that can delay the degradation or aid in the replenishment of dopamine may be prescribed. Medications may not benefit all patients. Surgery and deep brain stimulation is another treatment option when medications fail.

TOURETTE SYNDROME

- Also known as: Gilles de la Tourette syndrome

- Description: A neurological disorder characterized by repeated and uncontrolled involuntary movements and sounds ("tics"), which may include grunts, barks, or words (some words may be inappropriate). The condition is usually first noticed in childhood between the ages of 7 and 10 years. It occurs in all ethnic groups. Males are affected more than females. Although Tourette syndrome can be a chronic condition with symptoms lasting a lifetime, most people with the condition experience their worst symptoms in their early teens, with improvement occurring in the late teens and continuing into adulthood.

- Causes: Strong evidence exists suggesting that Tourette syndrome is an inherited condition passed on through generations.

- Clinical presentation
  - Arm thrusting
  - Eye blinking
  - Jumping
  - Kicking
  - Repeated throat clearing or sniffing
  - Shoulder shrugging
- Management: Treatment is not required unless the tics interfere with everyday life. Excitement or stress can exacerbate symptoms. Calm, focused activities help improve the disorder. Antipsychotic and antiepileptic medications are sometimes used to reduce the severity of symptoms. However, there is currently no medication that alleviates all symptoms, and not all medications work for all patients. Psychotherapy may help the patient better cope with the disorder and deal with the social and emotional issues that arise with the condition.

4

ENDOCRINE AND METABOLIC CONDITIONS

- Diabetes
  - Type 1 diabetes mellitus
  - Type 2 diabetes mellitus
- Hyperglycemia
- Hypoglycemia
- Polycystic ovary syndrome
- Thyroiditis
  - Hypothyroidism
  - Hyperthyroidism

Rehberg RS, Rehberg JS.
Cram Session in General Medical Conditions:
A Handbook for Students & Clinicians (pp. 49-64).
© 2012 Taylor & Francis Group.

DIABETES

- □ Also known as: Diabetes mellitus, insulin–dependent diabetes mellitus (Type 1 or juvenile onset), non-insulin–dependent diabetes mellitus (Type 2), brittle diabetes mellitus, endocrine diabetes mellitus, iatrogenic diabetes mellitus, latent diabetes mellitus, bronze diabetes, gestational diabetes, diabetes insipidus, pancreatic diabetes, phlorizin diabetes, renal diabetes

- □ Description: Common term for diseases characterized by extreme urination. The word diabetes is derived from the Greek verb *diabainein*, meaning to stand with legs apart (as if to urinate), or to pass through.

- □ Types of diabetes

  - o Diabetes mellitus—Disorder characterized by hyperglycemia and glycosuria resulting from inadequate production or utilization of insulin; failure of beta cells in the pancreas to supply the body's demand of insulin.

    - ■ Insulin–dependent diabetes mellitus (Type 1)—Caused by the body's insufficient production of insulin. Usually has its onset prior to the age of 25 (also known as juvenile onset diabetes).

    - ■ Non-insulin–dependent diabetes mellitus (Type 2)—Insulin produced by the pancreas is not enough to keep up with the body's demand because of the high levels of sugar build-up.

    - ■ Brittle diabetes mellitus—Unpredictable variation in a patient's glucose tolerance.

    - ■ Endocrine diabetes mellitus—A type of diabetes mellitus associated with diseases of the pituitary gland, thyroid gland, or adrenal gland.

    - ■ Iatrogenic diabetes mellitus—Diabetes mellitus caused by the administration of drugs such as corticosteroids, diuretics, or birth control pills.

    - ■ Latent diabetes mellitus—Type of diabetes mellitus that manifests during times of stress such as pregnancy, infectious disease, obesity, or trauma.

  - o Diabetic ketoacidosis (DKA)—Occurs when the body is unable to use glucose as a fuel source due to lacking or ineffective insulin. As a result, fat is broken down and used as a fuel source. Byproducts of the chemical breakdown of fat called ketones build up within the body. DKA is a medical emergency.

- o Bronze diabetes—Disease affecting metabolism of iron. Characteristics include enlargement of the liver, skin pigmentations of a bronzed hue, diabetes mellitus, and frequent cardiac failure.

- o Gestational diabetes—Diabetes that occurs for the first time during pregnancy.

- o Diabetes insipidus—Frequent passing of diluted urine because of its relatively low sodium content. Caused by a deficiency of vasopressin secretion by the pituitary gland or renal tubular unresponsiveness to vasopressin.

- o Pancreatic diabetes—A type of diabetes associated with pancreatic diseases.

- o Phlorizin diabetes—Administration of phlorizin produces renal glycosuria and blocks intestinal glucose.

- o Renal diabetes—Disorder characterized by a low renal threshold for sugar.

- □ Causes

  - o Damage to the pituitary gland, thyroid gland, and/or adrenal gland

  - o Failure of beta cells in the pancreas to secrete sufficient amounts of insulin to the body

  - o Caused by the body's resistance to insulin

- □ Clinical presentation

  - o Signs could include (but are not limited to):

    - ■ Dehydration

    - ■ High blood pressure

    - ■ Hypertension

    - ■ Hypotension

    - ■ Muscle atrophy

    - ■ Obesity

- Organ damage (severe)
- Skin turgor
- Ulcers
- Weight loss
- Yeast infections
- Boils and carbuncles
- Extreme fatigue and irritability
- Polyuria (frequent urination)
- Frequent or slow-healing infections
- Glycosuria
- Hyperglycemia
- Peripheral neuropathy
- Polydipsia (excessive thirst)
- Polyphagia (excessive hunger)
- Pruritus

☐ Management

  o Control of blood glucose

  o Diet management

  o Regular exercise

  o Insulin therapy

  o Low-dose aspirin

  o Medications

TYPE 1 DIABETES MELLITUS

☐ Also known as: Insulin–dependent diabetes mellitus, juvenile onset diabetes

☐ Description: A type of diabetes mellitus that usually starts prior to the age of 25 where carbohydrate, fat, and protein metabolisms fluctuate and are difficult to control due to insulin deficiency.

- Causes
  - Genetic inheritance
  - Damage to pancreatic beta cells from an infection
  - Environmental agents such as toxic chemicals, exposure to cow's milk during infancy, cytotoxins, and viral infections such as mumps and rubella can increase the risk of developing Type 1 diabetes mellitus.
- Clinical presentation
  - Altered mental status in some cases
  - Dehydration
  - Hypotension
  - Blurred vision
  - Ketoacidosis
  - Muscle cramping (due to electrolyte imbalance)
  - Nausea
  - Nocturnal enuresis (bedwetting)
  - Polydipsia
  - Polyphagia
  - Polyuria
  - Weight loss
- Management
  - Lifelong insulin therapy
  - Regular serum glucose monitoring
  - Complete retinal examination annually
  - An individualized comprehensive diet management that controls daily caloric intake and amounts of carbohydrate, fat, and protein intake
  - Regular exercise

- ❑ Other important information

  - ○ Type 1 diabetes mellitus is an autoimmune disease. It is a catabolic disorder in which the insulin circulating in the body is very low to none, plasma glucagon is high, and pancreatic beta cells do not respond to all insulin-secretory stimuli. Patients need an extreme amount of insulin to reverse this catabolic condition. Patients have an increased risk of developing heart diseases; cerebral vascular disease; peripheral vascular disease with gangrene of lower limbs; chronic renal disease; reduced visual acuity and blindness; and autonomic and peripheral neuropathy. This form of diabetes mellitus is usually quite difficult to regulate.

TYPE 2 DIABETES MELLITUS

- ❑ Also known as: Non-insulin–dependent diabetes mellitus

- ❑ Description: A type of diabetes mellitus that is usually diagnosed after age 45. In this form of diabetes, the pancreas secretes insulin; however, the body is unable to effectively use the insulin. This is often referred to as insulin resistance. Type 2 diabetes accounts for over 90% of diabetes cases.

- ❑ Causes and risk factors

  - ○ Ethnicity—African Americans, Native Americans, Hispanic Americans, and Japanese Americans are among the highest at risk

  - ○ Excessive alcohol consumption

  - ○ Genetic predisposition

  - ○ High-fat diet

  - ○ Hyperlipidemia

  - ○ Hypertension

  - ○ Increasing age

  - ○ Obesity

  - ○ Sedentary lifestyle

- ❑ Clinical presentation—symptom onset usually progresses gradually

  - ○ Blurred vision

  - ○ Dry mouth

- o Polyphagia
- o Polydipsia
- o Fatigue
- o Polyuria
- o Headache
- o Loss of consciousness
- o Weight loss
- □ Management
  - o Oral diabetes medications
  - o An individualized comprehensive diet management that controls daily caloric intake and amounts of carbohydrate, fat, and protein intake
  - o Regular exercise
  - o Insulin injection/pump
- □ Other important information
  - o Type 2 diabetes is no longer referred to as "adult onset" because the condition can occur in children and adolescents as well. Insulin injections may be necessary when oral medications and/or diet and exercise fail to adequately control the situation.

HYPERGLYCEMIA

- □ Description: A condition usually associated with diabetes in which excessive amounts of glucose circulates throughout the bloodstream. Two specific types of hyperglycemia include fasting hyperglycemia (90 to 130 mg/dL) or postprandial (after meal) hyperglycemia (180 mg/dL).
- □ Causes
  - o Decreased insulin levels due to skipping/missing injection
  - o Change in physical activity (increase or decrease)
  - o Failure to use glucose-lowering medication
  - o Increased or excessive caloric intake (especially carbohydrates)
  - o Stress

- Clinical presentation
  - Altered level of consciousness or coma
  - Blurred or decreased vision
  - Cardiac arrhythmia
  - Difficulty concentrating
  - Polyphagia
  - Polydipsia
  - Fatigue
  - Polyuria
  - Headache
  - Impotence
  - Infection
  - Poor wound healing
  - Stupor
  - Weight loss
- Hyperglycemia can be a result of acute DKA. Symptoms may include the following:
  - Acute hunger and thirst
  - Belligerence, confusion, and/or altered level of consciousness
  - Cognitive impairment
  - Deep, rapid breathing
  - "Fruity" or acetone odor on breath
  - Incontinence
- Management: Administration of insulin
- Other important information: Chronic hyperglycemia can lead to additional complications including cardiovascular, neurological, and retinal damage.

HYPOGLYCEMIA

- Description: Lower than normal blood glucose
- Causes
  - Improper regulation of blood glucose through insulin injection or medication in diabetics
  - Endocrine disorders
  - Excessive alcohol consumption
  - Fasting
  - Pancreatic tumor
  - Pre-existing illness
  - Poor diet
- Clinical presentation
  - Anxiety
  - Confusion and/or abnormal behavior
  - Diaphoresis
  - Hunger
  - Loss of consciousness
  - Seizures
  - Tremors
  - Visual disturbances
- Management
  - Management usually involves the administration of glucose:
    - If conscious and alert, consumption of candy, juice, or glucose tablets
    - If unconscious, use of glucose paste on the gums or sublingually
    - Use of glucagon injection kit (in severe episodes)
- Other important information: Hypoglycemia may occur as a complication of a diabetic condition. However, hypoglycemia can occur

in individuals who are not diabetic. Hypoglycemia may also occur after eating meals (called *postprandial hypoglycemia*) as a result of increased insulin production.

POLYCYSTIC OVARY SYNDROME

☐ Also known as: Stein-Leventhal syndrome

☐ Description: An endocrine disturbance associated with the presence of polycystic ovaries, hirsutism, and amenorrhea

☐ Causes: There is an increased stimulation of the ovarian theca cells due to increased stimulation of the luteinizing hormone, resulting in increased androgen production (testosterone and androstenedione). Due to the decreased stimulation of follicle-stimulating hormone relative to luteinizing hormone, the ovarian granulosa cells cannot convert the androgens to estrogens; hence, there is a decreased estrogen level and subsequent anovulation.

☐ Clinical presentation

　　o Acanthosis nigricans—A diffuse, velvety thickening and hyperpigmentation of the skin

　　o Alopecia

　　o Clitoromegaly

　　o Hirsutism—Excessive body hair and acne

　　o Hyperandrogenism—Excess terminal body hair in a male distribution pattern

　　o Increased muscle mass

　　o Increased serum blood levels for androgens

　　o Infertility

　　o Insulin resistance

　　o Menstrual abnormalities, including oligomenorrhea or amenorrhea

　　o Obesity

☐ Management: Goal is aimed at the treatment of anovulation, metabolic derangements, hirsutism, and irregular menstruation. Ultrasound imaging is often used to confirm diagnosis. Glucose tolerance testing may also be indicated.

□ Other important information: Consultation of an endocrinologist should be an option for further evaluations of biochemical and metabolic derangements. Consultation of a reproductive endocrinologist should be done for infertile patients who wish to become pregnant.

THYROIDITIS

□ Also known as: Acute suppurative thyroiditis, subacute thyroiditis, giant cell thyroiditis, chronic thyroiditis, Hashimoto's thyroiditis, microbial subacute thyroiditis, Riedel's thyroiditis, and invasive fibrous thyroiditis.

□ Description: Inflammation of the thyroid gland

   o Four types

      ■ Chronic or Hashimoto's thyroiditis—Autoimmune in nature, chronic thyroiditis is the most common inflammatory thyroid condition. It affects women 8 times more than men. It is commonly accompanied by the destruction of thyroid tissue due to lymphocytic infiltration.

      ■ Subacute or giant cell thyroiditis—Resulting from a viral infection of the thyroid gland, it usually follows a viral illness such as adenoviral infections, influenza, common cold, measles, mononucleosis, mumps, or myocarditis.

      ■ Acute suppurative thyroiditis (microbial subacute thyroiditis)— A rare form of thyroiditis resulting from a bacterial infection. Common bacteria responsible include *Staphylococcus aureus, Streptococcus hemolyticus,* and *pneumococcus.*

      ■ Invasive fibrosis or Riedel's thyroiditis—The most rare form of thyroiditis, characterized by fibrosis and resulting destruction of the thyroid gland.

□ Causes

   o Autoimmune deficiency

   o Bacterial infection

   o Viral infection

   o Iodine deficiency

   o Radiation therapy for head and neck cancers and lymphoma

- ☐ Clinical presentation
  - o Firm, enlarged thyroid gland
  - o The patient cannot tolerate palpation of the neck (severe)
  - o Goiter
  - o Fever
  - o Neck pain which radiates to the mandible, ears, or occiput
  - o Neck tenderness and swelling
  - o Neck flexion reduces the severity of the pain
  - o Neck hyperextension increases the severity of pain
  - o Fatigue
  - o Heat intolerance
  - o Increased nervousness
  - o Increased sweating
  - o Palpitations
  - o Tachycardia
- ☐ Management
  - o Acute suppurative thyroiditis
    - ▪ Requires immediate antibiotic therapy
  - o Subacute thyroiditis
    - ▪ Treatment goal is to relieve discomfort
    - ▪ Low-dose aspirin every 4 to 6 hours
    - ▪ Pharmacological treatment of patients who develop hypothyroidism
  - o Chronic thyroiditis
    - ▪ Dependent upon results of thyroid function tests
    - ▪ Pharmacological intervention may be used for patients with high thyroid stimulating hormone (TSH)
    - ▪ Often requires life-long thyroid hormone replacement therapy

- o Invasive fibrous thyroiditis

  - ▪ Often requires biopsy to rule out thyroid carcinoma

  - ▪ Surgical resection of thyroid may be indicated in symptomatic patients

- ☐ Other important information: Treatment of acute thyroiditis may require surgery to drain the abscess and correct developmental abnormalities. Patients with Down syndrome, Turner syndrome, Type 1 diabetes or other autoimmune or endocrine diseases are at risk for chronic thyroiditis. Chronic thyroiditis is the most common cause of goiter in the United States.

HYPOTHYROIDISM

- ☐ Description: Hypothyroidism is a common endocrine disorder resulting from deficiency of thyroid hormones T3 and T4.

- ☐ Causes

  - o Iodine deficiency (most common cause)

  - o Insufficient secretion of the thyroid gland

  - o Low basal metabolic rate

  - o Localized disease of the thyroid gland resulting in a decreased production of thyroid hormone

  - o Thyroid damage (from toxins, radiation)

- ☐ Clinical presentation

  - o Early signs and symptoms of hypothyroidism include the following:

    - ▪ Weight gain

    - ▪ Loss of hair

    - ▪ Goiter

    - ▪ Cold intolerance

    - ▪ Abdominal bloating

    - ▪ Loss or thinning of eyebrows

- Depression
- Decreased libido
- Muscle and/or joint pain
- Facial puffiness
- Ataxia
- Brittle nails
- Bradycardia
- Reduced cardiac output
- Dry skin
- Dull facial expression
- Jaundice
- Low blood pressure
- Pitting edema of lower extremities
- Slow speech and movements
- Blurred vision
- Decreased hearing
- Decreased sweating
- Hoarseness of voice
- Impaired memory
- Lethargy
- Obstructive sleep apnea
- Paresthesia and nerve entrapment syndromes
- Cold hands and feet

□ Management
  o Increase in iodine diet
  o Hormone replacement therapy

□ Other important information: Hypothyroidism is among the most common endocrine diseases. If untreated, hypothyroidism leads to myxedema (swelling and/or a waxy, coarse appearance of the skin and cheeks), coma, and/or death.

HYPERTHYROIDISM

□ Also known as: Thyrotoxicosis, Graves' disease

□ Description: Overactivity of the thyroid gland leading to disproportionate production of thyroid hormones and an increase in metabolism in the peripheral tissues

□ Causes

   o Excessive secretion of the thyroid gland

   o Increase in basal metabolic rate

   o Increase in the peripheral circulation of unbound thyroid hormones

□ Clinical presentation

   o Alterations in mental status

   o Anxiety

   o Diaphoresis

   o Diarrhea

   o Exaggerated deep-tendon reflexes

   o Heat intolerance

   o Hyperactivity

   o Hypertension

   o Hyperthermia

   o Increased circulation to the thyroid gland, causing thyroid bruit

   o Insomnia

   o Menstrual irregularities (females)

   o Muscle tremors

   o Muscle weakness

   o Ophthalmic pathology including exophthalmic goiter, periorbital edema, ophthalmoplegia, or optic atrophy

- o Palpitations
- o Symmetrical enlargement of the thyroid gland
- o Tachycardia
- o Weight loss
- ☐ Management
    - o Removal of the thyroid gland
    - o Use of antithyroid drugs such as propylthiouracil, methimazole, or carbimazole
    - o Use of beta-adrenergic blockade with propranolol
    - o Use of iodide
- ☐ Other important information: Hyperthyroidism is rare in children. Graves' disease, the most common form of hyperthyroidism, is 8 times more common in women than in men.

5

HEMATOLOGICAL AND ONCOLOGICAL CONDITIONS

- Anemia
  - Iron deficiency anemia
  - Sickle cell anemia
  - Vitamin B_{12} deficiency
  - Folate-deficiency anemia
  - Thalassemia
- Hemochromatosis
- Hemophilia A and B
- Leukemia
- Hodgkin's Lymphoma
- Non-Hodgkin's Lymphoma
- Multiple myeloma
- Prostate cancer
- Testicular cancer

Rehberg RS, Rehberg JS.
Cram Session in General Medical Conditions:
A Handbook for Students & Clinicians (pp. 65-82).
© 2012 Taylor & Francis Group.

- ☐ Colorectal cancer

- ☐ Lung cancer

- ☐ Breast cancer

- ☐ Bone cancer (primary bone tumors)

ANEMIA

- ☐ Description: A reduction in the number of red blood cells, or the amount of hemoglobin present in the blood is low. Red blood cells and hemoglobin are necessary for adequate transport of oxygen from the lungs to the rest of the body.

- ☐ Causes: See sickle cell anemia, B_{12} deficiency, folate deficiency, and beta-thalassemia conditions for additional or more specific information.

  - o Iron deficiency

  - o Cancer

  - o Chronic bleeding

  - o Folic acid deficiency

  - o Heavy menstrual cycle

  - o Pregnancy

  - o Chemotherapy

  - o Sudden excessive bleeding

  - o Vitamin B_{12} deficiency

  - o Decreased red blood cell production

  - o Increased red blood cell destruction

- ☐ Clinical presentation

  - o Fatigue

  - o Weakness

  - o Pallor

o Faintness

o Vertigo

o Increased thirst

o Irritability

o Sweating

o Weak rapid pulse and breathing

o Chest pain during exercise

☐ Management: See sickle cell anemia, B_{12} deficiency, folate deficiency, and beta-thalassemia conditions for additional or more specific information.

Anemia can be diagnosed using blood tests that measure the amount of hemoglobin and red blood cells in the blood. Treatment options depend on the cause of anemia but may include iron supplementation and treatment of chronic or bleeding disorders.

IRON DEFICIENCY ANEMIA

☐ Also known as: Athlete's anemia

☐ Description: Low levels of red blood cells as a result of inadequate levels of iron in the blood. Iron deficiency anemia is the most common form of anemia and can affect oxygen transport, DNA synthesis, electron transport, and growth and learning abilities in children. Iron levels are maintained through mucosal cells in the lining of the proximal small intestine.

☐ Causes

o Inadequate iron consumption

o Inability to absorb iron in the small intestine

o Hemorrhage

o Heavy bleeding during menstruation

o Excessive exercise—Excessive exercise can increase blood volume, and as a result, can cause an imbalance in the ratio between blood and iron. Known as athlete's anemia, normal blood volume and iron levels will return to normal usually within a week of normal physical activity.

◻ Clinical presentation

    ○ Brittle nails

    ○ Cyanosis

    ○ Decreased appetite

    ○ Fatigue

    ○ Headache

    ○ Irritability

    ○ Pallor

    ○ Shortness of breath

    ○ Tongue swelling and/or soreness

    ○ Pica (unusual food cravings)

    ○ Weakness

◻ Management: Depending on the cause, there are several treatment options for iron deficiency anemia, including oral supplementation of iron, a modified diet rich in iron, blood transfusions for chronic hemorrhage, and surgical repair of hemorrhage.

SICKLE CELL ANEMIA

◻ Also known as: Sickle cell disease

◻ Description: Sickle cell anemia is a genetically inherited disorder that affects the structure, shape, and productivity of hemoglobin in red blood cells. Sickle cell anemia is characterized by crescent-shaped red blood cells that, due to the abnormal shape, are unable to function normally. The red blood cells contain abnormal hemoglobin (termed *hemoglobin S*) and cause the red blood cell to become misshapen and stiff. The abnormal shape and rigidity of the cell's structure makes it difficult to pass through smaller blood vessels and can cause them to break apart. Excessive pain can be caused by oxygen deprivation due to blockage of blood flow in small vessels. Long term blockage of the vessels due to sickle cell can cause damage to the spleen, liver, kidneys, brain, and bones. Sickle cell crisis, or vaso-occlusive crisis, causes a sudden dramatic increase in symptoms, usually triggered by strenuous physical activity, flying at high altitudes, and mountain climbing where increased oxygen is consumed. Persons with sickle cell trait may be at increased risk for exertional rhabdomyolysis.

□ Causes: Sickle cell anemia is a genetically inherited disease affecting red blood cells and is most common in the African American, Native African, and Mediterranean populations.

□ Clinical presentation

   o Anemia

   o Jaundice

   o Difficulty breathing during strenuous activity

   o Chronic pain in the abdomen and long bones

   o Fatigue

   o Pallor

   o Scleral icterus

   o Splenomegaly

   o Heart murmurs

   o Leg ulcers

   o Weakness

□ Management: There is no cure for sickle cell anemia. However, interventions are available to aid in the management of specific symptoms. These include the following:

   o Pain control with the use of opioids as well as long-lasting oral doses of morphine for chronic pain

   o Prevention of infection with the use of various antibiotic treatments

   o Surgical care, such as skin grafts, to help heal leg ulcers

   o Folic acid supplementation to help aid in the production of red blood cells

VITAMIN B$_{12}$ DEFICIENCY

□ Also known as: Pernicious anemia

□ Description: A chronic condition caused by inadequate absorption of vitamin B$_{12}$ which is important for the formation of mature red blood cells, synthesis of DNA, and normal function of nerves.

- Causes: Most common cause of B_{12} deficiency is inadequate absorption due to a lack of intrinsic factor. Intrinsic factor is produced from the mucosal cells in the stomach and is required for vitamin B_{12} absorption. Inadequate levels of intrinsic factor cause vitamin B_{12} to pass through the intestines and excreted.

- Clinical presentation

  - Fatigue

  - Paleness

  - Shortness of breath

  - Vertigo

  - Weakness

- Severe cases

  - Confusion

  - Dementia

  - Difficulty walking

  - Loss of reflexes

  - Neurological dysfunction

  - Parasthesia in the extremities

  - Poor muscular function

- Management

  - Modification of diet to include Vitamin B_{12} rich foods

  - Oral vitamin supplementation

  - Intramuscular injections of vitamin B_{12}

FOLATE-DEFICIENCY ANEMIA

- Also known as: Folic acid deficiency, Megaloblastic anemia

- Description: A form of anemia resulting from inadequate levels of folic acid. Folic acid is a water soluble B vitamin found in green, leafy vegetables and the liver, which must be consumed daily in order to maintain proper blood levels. Folic acid is required for the production and growth of red blood cells. It also plays a role in DNA synthesis and in the use, breakdown, and production of proteins.

□ Causes

  o Alcoholism

  o Celiac disease

  o Eating overcooked food

  o Increased folate demand in women during pregnancy

  o Poor diet

  o Medications that affect the absorption of folate, such as phenytoin (Dilantin)

  o Surgical removal of portions of the stomach and/or small intestine, which is common in weight-loss surgery

□ Clinical presentation

  o Diarrhea

  o Fatigue

  o Graying of hair

  o Headache

  o Mouth and/or tongue ulcers

  o Pallor

  o Peptic ulcers

□ Management: Primary management includes the identification and treatment of the cause of the deficiency. Diet modification includes increased intake of leafy green vegetables and citrus fruits. Oral or intravenous folic acid supplements may be prescribed until the deficiency is corrected. In cases where absorption of folic acid is impaired (such as when following surgery), supplementation may be lifelong.

THALASSEMIA

□ Description: A group of hereditary anemias caused by an imbalance in the production of certain amino acids that make up hemoglobin. Thalassemias are classified as alpha-thalassemia, in which the alpha globin amino acid chain is affected; or beta-thalassemia, in which the beta globin chain is affected. Alpha-thalassemia is more common in African Americans, while beta-thalassemia is more common in individuals from the Mediterranean and Southeast Asia. Thalassemias are also classified based on whether 1 copy of the defective gene is present (known as thalassemia minor) or 2 copies are present (known as thalassemia major).

☐ Causes: Genetic dysfunction affecting the amino acid chains of hemoglobin

☐ Clinical presentation: Symptoms vary depending on the type of thalassemia. Individuals with alpha- and beta-thalassemia minor may not exhibit any symptoms.

  o Alpha-thalassemia major

    ▪ Fatigue

    ▪ Pallor

    ▪ Shortness of breath

    ▪ Splenomegaly

  o Beta-thalassemia major

    ▪ Gallstones

    ▪ Jaundice

    ▪ Skin ulcers

    ▪ Thickening of head and facial bones

    ▪ Weakening of long bones

    ▪ Delayed growth in children

    ▪ Delay in reaching puberty

☐ Management: Most individuals with minor thalassemias do not require treatment. In more severe (major) thalassemias, a bone marrow transplant may be required. Gene therapy is another treatment being studied; however, it has not yet proven effective.

HEMOCHROMATOSIS

☐ Also known as: Bronze diabetes

☐ Description: A hereditary disorder characterized by excessive absorption and accumulation of iron in various organs including the liver, pancreas, myocardial fibers, and other visceral cells. Hemochromatosis can be fatal, but in most cases it is treatable. Sometimes referred to as bronze diabetes due to a bronze pigmentation of the skin caused by excess iron levels, hemochromatosis is most common in White individuals of Northern European descent.

☐ Causes: Hereditary disease that causes a defect in the gene HFE

☐ Clinical presentation: Patients with hemochromatosis may be asymptomatic. Symptoms become more prevalent during middle age or later and most commonly affect women following menopause.

  o Abdominal pain

  o Abnormal bronze or gray pigmentation of the skin

  o Arthritis

  o Chronic fatigue

  o Damage to the adrenal glands

  o Diabetes mellitus

  o Early menopause

  o Heart abnormalities including arrhythmias and congestive heart failure

  o Impotence

  o Joint pain

  o Liver disease including an enlarged liver, cirrhosis, cancer, and liver failure

  o Thyroid disorders

  o Weakness

☐ Management: Hemochromatosis is diagnosed through genetic testing when a blood test shows elevated levels of iron, ferritin, and transferrin (iron transporters). Currently, phlebotomy (bloodletting) is the best course of treatment in order to remove excess iron from the blood. Depending on the severity of iron levels in the blood, up to a pint (500 mL) of blood will be removed once or twice a week for a duration ranging from a few months to a year. Annual blood testing is required in order to ensure proper levels of iron are being maintained in the bloodstream. Treatment success is high when the disease is recognized and treated before the organs are affected by the iron build-up.

HEMOPHILIA A AND B

☐ Also known as: Classic hemophilia (hemophilia A), Christmas disease (hemophilia B)

☐ Description: The most common severe bleeding disorder. It is deficiency of the coagulation factor VIII (hemophilia A) or factor IX (hemophilia B). Spontaneous hemarthrosis is the classic presentation of the disorder. It is sex-linked recessive and usually occurs in males; rarely females.

☐ Causes: Hemophilia is an inherited genetic disorder

☐ Clinical presentation: Easy bruising, nosebleeds, and hematuria. The severity of symptoms is inverse to amount of circulating levels of factor activity. With low levels (< 1%) there is spontaneous hemarthroses, most commonly affecting the knees, ankles, elbows, the muscles, and also the gastrointestinal tract. Profuse hemorrhage occurs with surgery or trauma. In mild cases (> 5%) spontaneous bleeding is uncommon and occurs only after trauma or surgery.

☐ Laboratory findings: Prolonged partial thromboplastin time (PTT); normal prothrombin time (PT), bleeding time, and fibrinogen levels

☐ Management: Replacement of factor VIII or IX concentrates

LEUKEMIA

☐ Description: A form of cancer affecting blood forming cells in bone marrow, where rapidly producing immature white blood cells accumulate within the blood and organs, resulting in increased vulnerability to infection, hemorrhage, and anemia.

☐ Causes: The exact cause of leukemia is unknown. However, several risk factors are believed to contribute to the development of leukemia. These include smoking, long-term exposure to certain chemicals, and exposure to radiation. Individuals who have an immediate family member with leukemia may have an increased risk.

- Clinical presentation

  o Constant infections

  o Enlarged lymph nodes

  o Fatigue

  o Fever, chills

  o Frequent infection

  o Localized or generalized lymphadenopathy

  o Night sweats

  o Splenomegaly

  o Weight loss

- Management: Management of leukemia is typically a 2-pronged approach: treatment for the relief of symptoms and treatment of the cancer itself. Chemotherapy is typically used to treat the cancer, and may be administered via oral or intravenous medication. During chemotherapy, treatment may also include antibiotics and other drugs that prevent infection and the production of healthy red blood cells. Stem cell transplantation may also be used in conjunction with chemotherapy. Radiation therapy may also be used to treat some forms of the disease. Side effects such as hair loss, nausea, vomiting, sores of the mouth and tongue, loss of appetite, and low serum blood counts may be caused by chemotherapy.

HODGKIN'S LYMPHOMA

- Description: A form of cancer that affects the immune system, characterized by a large multinucleated cell known as Reed-Sternberg. This form of lymphoma can affect persons of all ages; however, it is most common among individuals aged 15 to 35 and patients age 50 and older. It usually forms in the lymph tissue of the lymph nodes, liver, spleen, and bone marrow. Most cases of Hodgkin's lymphoma are curable.

- Causes: The cause for Hodgkin's lymphoma is unknown. However, there is a connection between Hodgkin's lymphoma and Epstein-Barr virus, as approximately half of all Hodgkin's patients test positive for Epstein-Barr.

- Clinical presentation: Patients with Hodgkin's lymphoma often notice 1 or more enlarged lymph nodes, usually in the neck, groin, or armpit. Other signs and symptoms include the following:

  - Fatigue

  - Fever

  - Muscle weakness

  - Night sweats

  - Shortness of breath

  - Swollen, painless lymph nodes

  - Weight loss

- Management: Blood tests can be used to detect the presence of Reed-Sternberg cells. Chest x-ray, computed tomography (CT) scan, and positron emission tomography (PET) scan may also be used to confirm diagnosis and determine the stage of cancer. Treatment options such as chemotherapy and radiation therapy have a high success rate. Side effects such as hair loss, nausea, vomiting, sores of the mouth and tongue, loss of appetite, and low serum blood counts may be caused by chemotherapy.

NON-HODGKIN'S LYMPHOMA

- Also known as: Lymphoma, NHL

- Description: Non-Hodgkin's lymphoma is a cancer that affects the immune system. It can affect either B-lymphocytes or T-lymphocytes, which are the cells responsible for defending against bacteria, viruses, and fungi. Non-Hodgkin's lymphoma alters these cells, impairing their ability to fight infection. Non-Hodgkin's lymphoma is measured in stages (I, II, III, and IV) and is most severe in the fourth stage, where it attacks bone marrow and disrupts various blood cells in the body.

- Causes: In most cases, there is no definitive cause, although a weakened immune system may predispose a person to non-Hodgkin's lymphoma. Epstein-Barr virus has also been associated with lymphoma.

☐ Clinical presentation: The primary symptom of lymphoma is often enlarged, painless lymph nodes in the neck, groin, and armpits. Other symptoms may include the following:

o Difficulty breathing

o Fatigue

o Fever

o Night sweats

o Loss of appetite

o Red patches on the skin

o Weight loss

☐ Management: Lymph node and bone marrow biopsies are used to diagnose non-Hodgkin's lymphoma. Blood chemistry tests, CT, and PET scans are also used to confirm diagnosis and stage. In the earlier stages of non-Hodgkin's lymphoma, chemotherapy and radiation therapy have proven effective in curing the cancer. Antibiotics are given in order to help the body fend off viruses and infections. Later stages (stage IV) of non-Hodgkin's lymphoma affect the bone marrow, which further disrupts cell count of red blood cells, white blood cells, and platelets. Patients who are in stage IV of non-Hodgkin's lymphoma have a low level of success with treatment. However, most people are cured or have long survival rates. Side effects such as hair loss, nausea, vomiting, sores of the mouth and tongue, loss of appetite, and low serum blood counts may be caused by chemotherapy.

MULTIPLE MYELOMA

☐ Description: Multiple myeloma is a form of cancer characterized by abnormal plasma cells in the bone marrow. Typically, plasma cells make up 1% of bone marrow; in multiple myeloma, the amount of abnormal plasma cells impede the normal function of bone marrow, preventing the production of red blood cells, white blood cells, and platelets. The abundance of cancerous plasma cells eventually form a tumor (plasmacytoma) which leads to the breakdown of bone, causing osteoporosis most commonly in the pelvis, spine, ribs, and skull. The breakdown of bone causes an increased level of calcium in the blood, resulting in additional health concerns. Multiple myeloma accounts for 1% of all cancers.

- Causes: No definitive cause has been determined; however, heredity and exposure to radiation may play a role.

- Clinical presentation

  - Anemia

  - Bone pain

  - Bone fractures, especially of the spine, pelvis, ribs, and skull

  - Appearance of "punched out" bone defects on radiographic imaging

  - Elevated calcium levels which may lead to constipation, persistent urination, and weakness

  - Kidney dysfunction

  - Immunocompromised

  - Increased infections

  - Shortness of breath

  - Weakness and fatigue

- Management: Blood chemistry and urinalysis can be used to detect "M" protein, which is produced by myeloma cells. Definitive diagnosis is made through bone marrow biopsy. Several different treatment options exist. Treatment often includes chemotherapy as well as the use of corticosteroids, immunomodulating agents, and stem cell transplantation. Side effects such as hair loss, nausea, vomiting, sores of the mouth and tongue, loss of appetite, and low serum blood counts may be caused by chemotherapy.

PROSTATE CANCER

- Description: Cancer of the prostate gland. The most common cancer detected in American men.

- Risk factors: Age (diagnosis is rare before age 40; most cases diagnosed in males aged 50 or older), ethnicity (occurs most often in African-American men), family history, genetic predisposition, obesity, smoking, and diet rich in meat and dairy products

- Clinical presentation: Cancer is most often asymptomatic. It is usually detected upon digital rectal exam with finding of nodule or areas of induration within the prostate, or with elevation of prostate-specific antigen (PSA). Symptoms may include urinary retention, painful urination, blood in the urine, weight loss, and bone pain. The diagnosis of prostate cancer is confirmed with prostatic biopsy.

□ Management: Treatment is determined according to TNM cancer staging and grade: T for primary tumor, N for regional lymph nodes, and M for distant metastasis. Grading is based on architectural criteria; there are 5 possible grades. Treatments include radical prostatectomy, radiation therapy, hormone therapy, and cryotherapy. In some individuals, no treatment is initiated and PSA levels are monitored.

TESTICULAR CANCER

□ Description: Cancer of the testis. It is the most common malignancy in males between the ages of 15 to 35.

□ Risk factors: Family history, human immunodeficiency virus (HIV) infection, age (most cases diagnosed in men aged 20 to 55), cryptorchidism, and ethnicity (White males are believed to be at highest risk).

□ Clinical presentation: The most common symptom is a painless, enlarging testicular mass. Scrotal ultrasound is performed to evaluate the mass. Tumor markers used for the diagnosis and treatment of testicular cancer are alpha-fetoprotein, human chorionic gonadotropin (hCG), and lactate dehydrogenase (LDH).

□ Management: Diagnosis is made via testicular biopsy. Chest x-ray and CT scan of the abdomen and pelvis are performed to determine staging of the disease. Treatment can include chemotherapy, radiation, and radical orchiectomy.

COLORECTAL CANCER

□ Description: Cancer of the colon (large intestine) or rectum. It is the second leading cause of death among Americans. It is more common in individuals older than 50 years of age. Most colorectal cancers arise from adenomatous polyps.

□ Risk factors: Risk factors include age, family history, personal history, inflammatory bowel disease, a diet rich in fat and low in fiber, smoking, and obesity.

- Clinical presentation: In the initial stages, colorectal cancer may be asymptomatic. Colorectal screening should be performed annually after age 50 and in individuals with a personal or family history. Screening includes fecal occult blood testing, sigmoidoscopy, and colonoscopy. Common symptoms include colicky abdominal pain, change in bowel habits, weakness and fatigue from anemia, unexplained weight loss, and blood in or on the stool.

- Management: Treatment is determined according to cancer staging. Polyps found during routine screening with colonoscopy can be removed. Surgery is needed for larger tumors. Radiation and chemotherapy may be needed for advanced cancers.

LUNG CANCER

- Description: Lung cancer is the leading cause of cancer death among men and woman, most commonly presenting between the ages of 50 and 70. The majority of cancers can be classified into two groups: non-small cell and small cell. Non-small cell is composed of adenocarcinomas, squamous cell, and large cell. Rarer types include mesothelioma, sarcomas, and carcinoid tumors.

- Causes: Cigarette smoking is the leading cause of lung cancer. Other causes include secondhand smoke, asbestos, ionizing radiation, and industrial carcinogens.

- Clinical presentation: Most patients (75% to 90%) are symptomatic at the time of diagnosis. Symptoms vary according to the position of the tumor, metastases, systemic effects, and coexisting paraneoplastic syndromes. Symptoms include cough, hemoptysis, chest pain, and shortness of breath. Anemia, weight loss, lymphadenopathy, hepatomegaly, and clubbing can also be present in patients with lung cancer.

- Diagnosis: Chest x-ray demonstrates abnormal findings. Old and new x-ray comparison can reveal characteristics suggestive of the different types of cancer, and add in the prognostication of the disease. CT scan, magnetic resonance imaging (MRI), and ultrasound can also be used to determine the extent of the tumor, evaluation of surrounding tissue, and in guiding therapeutic options. The diagnosis of lung cancer is made from cytologic examination via sputum, bronchoscopy, needle biopsy, and rarely mediastinoscopy and mediastinotomy.

- Management: The treatment of lung cancer includes surgery, chemotherapy, and therapy. Treatment is based on the cell type and staging of the cancer.

Cancer staging of lung cancer is according to tumor size (T), regional lymph node involvement (N), and distant metastases (M). TMN categories are further grouped into 4 stages.

BREAST CANCER

□ Description: Cancer of the breast tissue. Most commonly occurs in females but can occur in males as well. Breast cancer is the second leading cause of death from cancer among women.

□ Risk factors: The exact cause of breast cancer is not known; however, risk factors include inherited and acquired gene mutations, age (median age of diagnosis is 60 to 61), family history, exposure to radiation, race (Caucasian females appear to be at highest risk), increased breast density, and obesity.

□ Clinical presentation: Can be asymptomatic. Initial signs are abnormal mammography and palpable breast lump, which may or may not be painful. Axillary swelling, noticeable change in the appearance of the breast and/or nipple, and nipple discharge may be present. Later signs include nipple retraction, pain, swelling, and redness of the breast, as well as fixation of the mass to chest wall.

□ Management: Screening should begin at age 40 and include self-breast exam, clinical breast exam, and mammography; further testing may include ultrasound, breast MRI, and biopsy. Screening should begin sooner in high-risk individuals: women with a mother or sister with breast cancer, presence of breast cancer 1 (BRCA1) or BRCA2 mutation, previous medical history of endometrial cancer or cancer of the other breast, early menarche (age 12) or late menopause (age 50), nulliparity, or late first pregnancy.

Breast cancer staging determines the extent of treatment. Therapies include surgery—either lumpectomy or mastectomy—radiation therapy, chemotherapy, hormone therapy, and biological therapy. TNM staging of breast cancer is determined according to tumor size (T), regional lymph node involvement (N), and distant metastases (M). TNM categories are further grouped into 4 stages.

BONE CANCER (PRIMARY BONE TUMORS)

- Also known as: Osteosarcoma, Ewing's sarcoma, chondrosarcoma

- Description

  - Osteosarcoma—Primary bone tumor arising from osteoblasts. It is the most common malignant bone tumor in youth with an average age of 15. It typically presents during periods of most rapid bone growth. Males and females are equally affected until age 13, when males are predominantly affected. The most commonly affected bones are the tibia, femur, and humerus. Tumors typically occur in the long bones at the areas of fastest growth, the growth plates. The most common site of metastasis is to the lung. CT scan of the chest is recommended to determine if pulmonary metastasis has occurred.

  - Ewing's sarcoma—A primary malignant bone tumor with unknown cell origin. The average age of those affected is 15 years; it primarily affects individuals during periods of rapid growth. Males and females are equally affected until 13 years of age.

  - Chondrosarcoma—A primary malignant bone tumor arising from cartilage cells. It is the second most common bone sarcoma. Incidence increases with age; the peak incidence is the sixth or seventh decade. Chondrosarcomas often affect the axial skeleton.

- Clinical presentation: Symptoms include pathologic bone fractures, bone pain, swelling, and limited motion. Weight loss, fever, and malaise may also occur. Radiographs reveal bony deformities, densities, or lucencies. MRI reveals extent of local tumor. Biopsy reveals histologic evidence of bone neoplasm.

- Management: Chemotherapy and surgical excision

6

GASTROINTESTINAL AND HEPATIC/BILIARY CONDITIONS

- ☐ Acute pancreatitis
- ☐ Celiac disease
- ☐ Cholecystitis
- ☐ Constipation
- ☐ Diverticular disease
- ☐ Dyspepsia
- ☐ Gastroenteritis
- ☐ Hepatitis
- ☐ Hemorrhoids
- ☐ Hiatal hernia
- ☐ Peptic ulcer disease
- ☐ Irritable bowel syndrome
- ☐ Crohn's disease
- ☐ Gastroesophageal reflux disease
- ☐ Ulcerative colitis

Rehberg RS, Rehberg JS.
Cram Session in General Medical Conditions:
A Handbook for Students & Clinicians (pp. 83-102).
© 2012 Taylor & Francis Group.

ACUTE PANCREATITIS

- ❑ Description: An acute inflammation of the pancreas which occurs when the pancreatic enzymes become active within the pancreas rather than in the duodenum. The active enzymes self-digest the pancreatic cells, which in turn causes an inflammatory response. Pain usually begins in the upper epigastric area and gradually intensifies and becomes more consistent. Acute pancreatitis can be a severe, life-threatening condition.

- ❑ Causes

  - o Biliary tract disease secondary to gallstones

  - o Alcoholism

  - o Blunt trauma

  - o Illicit drug use

  - o Viral infections

  - o Bacterial infections

- ❑ Clinical presentation: The most common symptom is severe abdominal pain in the upper abdomen, right below the sternum. Other signs and symptoms include the following:

  - o Nausea

  - o Vomiting

  - o Referred pain to the back and/or left shoulder

  - o Anorexia

  - o Diarrhea

  - o Fever

  - o Tachycardia

  - o Abdominal tenderness, distension, and muscular guarding

- ❑ Management: Diagnostic tests including abdominal ultrasound, computed tomography (CT) scan, and magnetic resonance cholangiopancreatography (MRCP) are often used to confirm the diagnosis. Typically, patients are hospitalized and must fast for 2 to

3 days in order to rest the pancreas. Treatment typically includes analgesic medications, IV fluids, and antibiotics. Patients are slowly reintroduced to a normal diet consisting of low-fat foods and clear liquids. Severe acute pancreatitis requires the patient to be placed in intensive care where the vitals, blood levels, and urine production are closely monitored. Acute pancreatitis resulting from gallstones may require surgical removal of the stones if they are not passed.

CELIAC DISEASE

- Description: Inflammatory damage to the small intestinal mucosa, resulting from ingestion of gluten. Gluten is a storage protein in grains such as wheat, rye, and barley. The result is malabsorption of certain nutrients—carbohydrates, fats, electrolytes, proteins, calcium, magnesium, iron, zinc, folate, and fat-soluble vitamins. Mechanism of damage is not understood, though it is thought to be an immune response associated with human leukocyte antigen (HLA) class II antigens to gluten that causes intestinal inflammation. Clinically presents in infancy, but occasionally in the second to fourth decades.

- Causes: Genetic predisposition

- Clinical presentation: Symptoms vary depending on the severity of intestinal involvement.

  - Significant mucosal involvement

    - Watery diarrhea

    - Flatulence

    - Weight loss

    - Weakness

    - Growth retardation

  - Proximal intestine involvement

    - Anemia

    - Osteopenia or osteoporosis

  - Extraintestinal manifestations include the following:

    - Dermatitis herpetiformis

    - Peripheral neuropathy

- Depression

- Paranoia

- Infertility

- Spontaneous abortion

- Short stature

- Cardiomyopathy

□ Laboratory findings: Abnormalities vary depending on intestinal involvement; some may present with microcytic anemia due to iron deficiency, megaloblastic anemia due to folate deficiency, and low serum calcium.

□ Management: Diagnosis can be made if improvement is seen with introduction of a gluten-free diet. Definitive diagnosis is made with positive serologic markers and/or from intestinal biopsy. Most patients will experience improvement with the introduction of a gluten-free diet. Affected individuals should be screened for osteopenia/osteoporosis and for vitamin and mineral deficiencies.

CHOLECYSTITIS

□ Also known as: Gallbladder disease, gallbladder attack

□ Description: An inflammation of the gallbladder, most commonly caused by a blockage of the cystic duct. The inflammation of the gallbladder occurs from the build-up of bile due to the blockage. Cholecystitis can be acute or chronic. Acute cholecystitis occurs following major surgery, serious illness or infection, intravenous feedings or fasting for an extended period of time, or an immune system deficiency. Chronic cholecystitis occurs as a result of repeated gallstones (cholelithiasis) causing the tissues to become thickened and scarred. Factors that increase risk of gallstones include age (patients aged 40 and older are at greater risk), obesity, a high-cholesterol diet, and gender (females are at a higher risk due to estrogen levels).

□ Causes

o Cardiac pathology, including myocardial infarction

o Critical illness

- o   Diabetes mellitus

- o   Major burns

- o   Major surgery

- o   Prolonged fasting

- o   Prolonged intravenous feedings

- o   Salmonella infections

- o   Sepsis

- o   Sickle cell disease

□   Clinical presentation

- o   Pain that lasts longer than 6 hours

- o   Belching

- o   Constipation

- o   Diarrhea

- o   Enlarged, palpable gallbladder

- o   Fever

- o   Heartburn

- o   Intolerance of spicy or fatty foods

- o   Jaundice

- o   Referred pain in right shoulder

- o   Right upper quadrant tenderness

- o   Vomiting

□   Management: Acute cholecystitis treatment includes bowel rest, IV fluids and nutrition, analgesics for pain management, and IV antibiotics. In acute cholecystitis, the gallbladder is usually removed 24 to 48 hours after onset of symptoms. In chronic cholecystitis, the gallbladder is removed after the acute attack resolves.

CONSTIPATION

- Description: A decrease in frequency (3 times or fewer per week) in passing stool or difficulty releasing bowel movements, which results from straining to release the stool, a hard sensation of one's stool, or the sensation of incomplete bowel movements.

- Causes
  - Poor diet (high sugar, low fiber)
  - Dehydration
  - Medications
  - Stress
  - Inactivity
  - Left colon obstruction
  - Outlet obstruction
  - Gastrointestinal disease

- Clinical presentation
  - Difficulty in passing of stool
  - Increased hardening of stool
  - Increased size of stool
  - Abdominal discomfort
  - Tearing of anus due to increase size of stool

- Management: Initial treatment includes increasing the amount of fiber and hydration. Exercise is also recommended to help with bowel movements. Laxatives, suppositories, and enemas may be recommended if other management is not successful.

- Additional information: Constipation can be a sign of other serious illness. Changes in bowel movement frequency should be evaluated by a physician.

DIVERTICULAR DISEASE

- Also known as: Diverticulosis, diverticulitis

❑ Description: Diverticular disease is characterized by small herniations, sacs known as diverticula, that protrude through the mucosa, submucosa, or the entire thickness of the muscular wall. Although the sigmoid is the most commonly affected area, the disease may occur in the descending, ascending, and transverse sections of the colon and also in the jejunum, ileum, and duodenum. If the diverticula become inflamed, the disease is known as diverticulitis.

❑ Causes

   o High-fat and beef diets

   o Diets low in fiber

   o Colonic motility disorders

   o Corticosteroid therapy

   o Colonic segmentation

   o Defects in colonic wall strength

❑ Clinical presentation

   o Abdominal pain (usually on the left side)

   o Constipation

   o Diarrhea

   o Dysuria (if bladder is irritated)

   o Flatulence

   o High fever

   o Localized tenderness

   o Muscular guarding

   o Nausea

   o Rebound tenderness

   o Severe back and lower extremity pain

   o Vomiting

❑ Management: A high-fiber diet and light exercise to encourage bowel movement is the most common treatment. Surgery and antibiotic therapy may be required in more severe cases involving complete bowel obstruction or infection.

DYSPEPSIA

- □ Also known as: Heartburn, indigestion

- □ Description: Dyspepsia is the most common upper gastroenterological condition and is characterized by discomfort or a burning sensation in the epigastric region resulting from an irritation of the esophageal mucosum by gastric acid reflux.

- □ Causes
  - o Stomach ulcers
  - o Duodenal ulcers
  - o Stomach cancer
  - o Gastritis
  - o Gallstones lodged in the bile duct
  - o Aspirin and other nonsteroidal anti-inflammatory drugs (NSAID) use
  - o Alcohol
  - o Caffeine
  - o Pregnancy

- □ Clinical presentation
  - o Belching
  - o Burning sensation in the epigastric region
  - o Constipation
  - o Diarrhea
  - o Flatulence
  - o Increase or decrease in pain with eating
  - o Loud intestinal signs
  - o Nausea
  - o Poor appetite

- Management: Antacids are often used for relief of symptoms. In more severe cases, proton pump inhibitors or histamine 2 (H2) blockers may be more effective. If these treatments are unsuccessful, endoscopy may be necessary.

GASTROENTERITIS

- Also known as: Stomach flu, food poisoning, traveler's diarrhea

- Description: An inflammation of the lining of the stomach or small and large intestines caused by an infection from a microorganism or due to the ingestion of a chemical toxin or drug. Gastroenteritis may also be caused by a virus (known as the stomach flu), or bacteria (*Escherichia coli*).

- Causes

  o There are 4 categories of viruses that can cause gastroenteritis:

    - Rotavirus (the leading cause of gastroenteritis in children)

    - Calicivirus (predominantly the norovirus, found in contaminated water)

    - Astrovirus

    - Adenovirus (found in fecal-oral transmission)

  o Bacterial causes include

    - *E coli*

    - Shigella

    - Salmonella

    - Campylobacter

  o Parasites

  o Chemical toxins

- Clinical presentation

  o Abdominal cramping

  o Audible noises of the intestine

  o Dehydration

- o Diarrhea

- o Distended abdomen

- o Extreme exhaustion

- o Fever

- o Flu-like symptoms

- o Loss of appetite

- o Muscle aches

- o Nausea

- o Visible blood and/or mucous in stool

- o Vomiting

□ Management: The most common treatment is bed rest and the consumption of fluids. If vomiting and diarrhea continue and dehydration worsens, IV fluids and electrolytes may be necessary. Antiemetic drugs may be given to adults to control vomiting but are not recommended for children. As the symptoms subside, bland foods may be slowly added back into the diet. Prevention of traveler's diarrhea includes avoiding unprocessed foods and beverages (including water), and prophylactic vaccinations when traveling to certain geographic regions.

HEPATITIS

□ Also known as: Hepatitis A, B, C, D, E; toxic hepatitis; chronic or acute hepatitis

□ Description: An inflammation of the liver that is usually the result of a viral infection or liver toxicity. Hepatitis can be acute or chronic. Cases range from mild to life-threatening. There are several forms of hepatitis, including the following:

- o Hepatitis A: An RNA virus transmitted via oral-to-oral or fecal-to-oral route. Most commonly contracted via contaminated food or water and often due to improper or unsanitary food preparation. Incubation period is approximately 2 to 6 weeks; acute stage lasts approximately 2 to 12 weeks.

- o Hepatitis B: A DNA virus transmitted via exposure to infected blood or other potentially infectious materials (saliva, urine, feces, mucus, tears, vomit, semen, or vaginal secretions). Incubation period is 2 to 6 months. Acute infection usually resolves in 6 months. IV drug abusers, individuals with multiple sex partners, and health care workers are at greatest risk for transmission.

- o Hepatitis C: An RNA virus transmitted via exposure to infected blood or other potentially infectious materials (saliva, urine, feces, mucus, tears, vomit, semen, or vaginal secretions). Incubation period is approximately 6 to 12 weeks, and the acute phase lasts approximately 4 weeks. IV drug abusers, individuals with multiple sex partners, and health care workers are at greatest risk for transmission.

- o Hepatitis D: An RNA virus which causes infection only when hepatitis B virus is present. Also known as delta hepatitis.

- o Hepatitis E: An RNA virus similar to hepatitis A.

- o Toxic hepatitis: Caused by ingestion or absorption of toxic chemicals, including anabolic steroids.

- □ Clinical presentation: Depending on stage and severity, one or more of the following signs and symptoms may be present in individuals with hepatitis:

  - o Diarrhea

  - o Fatigue

  - o Hematuria

  - o Hepatomegaly, tender upon palpation

  - o Jaundice

  - o Joint pain

  - o Loss of appetite

  - o Nausea

  - o Swollen lymph nodes

  - o Weight loss

☐ Management: Prevention is the best method of management, including practicing infection control in healthcare settings, washing hands when working with food, limiting the amount of objects or foods that one shares with another person, and by using a condom during sex. The hepatitis B vaccine is effective in protecting against hepatitis B and D. Hepatitis A usually resolves without treatment over several weeks. Acute hepatitis B usually resolves without treatment, while the chronic hepatitis B and hepatitis C is treated with alpha interferon and peginterferon. Severe cases of hepatitis B may be treated with antiviral drugs. Chronic hepatitis D is treated with pegylated interferon. Hepatitis E normally resolves on its own over a period of several weeks or months.

HEMORRHOIDS

☐ Also known as: Piles, internal hemorrhoids, external hemorrhoids

☐ Description: Hemorrhoids are characterized by dilated or twisted varicose veins that are located in the rectum or the anus. Increased pressure within the veins causes them to become inflamed. This pressure usually causes lumps to form on the inside and/or outside of the anus, leading to pain and/or bleeding during defecation. External hemorrhoids are those that form below the anorectal junction. Hemorrhoids that form above the anorectal junction are called internal hemorrhoids.

☐ Causes: Increased pressure in the veins of the area between the anus and rectum can cause hemorrhoids. This pressure can derive from:

   o Pregnancy

   o Genetic predisposition

   o Holding one's breath during heavy lifting

   o Repeated straining or "bearing down" during bowel movements

☐ Clinical presentation

   o External hemorrhoids

      ▪ Painful, swollen lumps on the anus

      ▪ Pain and itching, usually while sitting

- o Internal hemorrhoids

    - Bleeding during defecation
    - Pain during defecation

- Management: Hemorrhoids are not usually medically serious and are treated with changes in diet, stool softeners, soaking the anus in warm water, and topical medications to relieve symptoms. Bleeding hemorrhoids can be treated with injection. Larger hemorrhoids may be removed using a procedure called rubber band ligation. The bands are tied around the hemorrhoids, causing them to drop off painlessly within 2 weeks. Internal hemorrhoids can be removed using laser therapy, infrared light, or electrical current. Surgical removal of hemorrhoids is considered as a last resort and can be painful.

HIATAL HERNIA

- Also known as: Sliding hiatal hernia, paraesophageal hiatal hernia

- Description: A protrusion of part of the proximal stomach through the esophageal hiatus (an opening in the diaphragm through which the esophagus passes). As a result, lower esophageal sphincter function is impaired, often producing backflow of stomach contents into the esophagus. There are 2 types of a hiatal hernia: sliding hiatal hernia (most common), where the gastroesophageal junction and the stomach are displaced above the diaphragm; or paraesophageal hiatus hernia, where the gastroesophageal junction remains in place, but the stomach is pushed above the diaphragm, next to the esophagus.

- Causes: Causes of this disorder are not usually known; however, age (more common in patients age 50 and older), obesity, and smoking are all known risk factors for acquiring hiatal hernia. Hiatal hernias are more common in women due to the intra-abdominal forces exerted during pregnancy.

- Clinical presentation

    - o Belching

    - o Bloating

    - o Chest pain

    - o Difficulty swallowing

o Indigestion

o Reflux

Symptoms worsen while supine due to acid flow into the esophagus.

□ Management: Diagnosis is confirmed through an upper GI series with barium x-ray. The treatment goal is to relieve symptoms. Medications to reduce stomach acidity or decrease acid production may be indicated. Behavior modification including eating small meals, weight loss, smoking cessation, and eliminating consumption of food and fluids that increase acid production—including alcohol, coffee, chocolate, onions, peppers, spices, and fatty foods—may be recommended. Surgical removal of a paraesophageal hiatal hernia may be required to prevent strangulation.

PEPTIC ULCER DISEASE

□ Also known as: PUD

□ Description: A lesion (ulcer) of the lining of the duodenum, lower esophagus, or stomach usually caused by an increase in gastric acid or an imbalance in the mucosal layer. Ulcers are named by the location affected or by the conditions under which they develop. duodenal ulcers (the most common) occur in the first few inches of the duodenum. Gastric ulcers usually occur in the upper curvature of the stomach. Stress ulcers can result from stress or severe illness or trauma. Lastly, marginal ulcers may develop following surgical removal of part of the stomach. Risk of peptic ulcers increases with age.

□ Causes

o Infection of the stomach with *Helicobacter pylori* bacteria

o Chronic use of NSAIDs

o Alcohol abuse

o Nicotine use

o Psychological and physiological stress

□ Clinical presentation

o Abdominal pain at night

o Intermittent pain in the upper and middle abdomen

- o Loss of appetite

- o Pain radiating from abdomen to the thoracic spine, chest, and neck

- o Pain that worsens or improves after eating

- o Vomiting

- o Weight loss

- □ Management: Avoidance of foods that irritate the ulcer. Antacids can be used to provide relief of symptoms. Drugs such as sucralfate may be used to form a protective coating in the base of the ulcer to promote healing. Prophylactic medications may also be indicated to reduce the likelihood of additional ulcers developing. Antibiotics may also be prescribed to control *H pylori*. Surgical intervention is usually not indicated.

IRRITABLE BOWEL SYNDROME

- □ Also known as: IBS, spastic colon, irritable colon, nervous colon

- □ Description: A digestive tract disorder characterized by abdominal pain, abnormal bowel habits, and inflammation of the bowels

- □ Causes: There is no definitive cause of IBS. Patients experience exacerbations of the condition for different reasons, which include the following:

  - o Emotional factors (stress, anxiety, and depression)

  - o Diet

  - o Medication

  - o Hormones

  - o High-calorie diets

  - o Diets high in fat, wheat, dairy products, coffee, tea, nicotine, alcohol, and citrus fruits are known to cause exacerbations of IBS

  - o Eating too quickly or waiting too long in between meals can also cause exacerbations of IBS

- □ Clinical presentation

  - o Abdominal distention with the build-up of gas

  - o Abdominal pain during bowel movement

- o Abdominal pain relieved by bowel movement

- o Bloating

- o Constipation

- o Diarrhea

- o Fatigue

- o Feeling of incomplete defecation

- o Headaches

- o Nausea

- □ Management: The most common treatments are stress reduction, dietary changes, and an increase in physical activity. Prescription and over-the-counter medication—such as anticholinergics, GI motility enhancers, antidiarrheal medications, and laxatives—may be indicated. IBS triggers such as alcohol, nicotine, caffeine, and others should be avoided.

CROHN'S DISEASE

- □ Also known as: Inflammatory bowel disease, regional enteritis, granulomatous ileitis, ileocolitis

- □ Description: A chronic inflammatory bowel disease characterized by patches of inflammation along areas of the digestive tract. Complications from inflammation can lead to fibrosis and obstruction. Although Crohn's disease can affect any part of the digestive tract, it most commonly affects the terminal aspect of the ileum and the proximal large intestine.

- □ Causes: Crohn's disease is idiopathic in nature. However, potential risk factors include genetics, impaired immune system, diet, and environmental factors. Smoking, use of NSAIDs, and oral contraceptives are also potential risk factors.

- □ Clinical presentation

- o Abdominal cramps

- o Abdominal pain

- o Chronic diarrhea

- o Fever

o Loss of appetite

o Stool containing mucus or blood

o Weight loss

o Impaired growth (in children)

☐ Management: There is no cure for Crohn's disease. The treatment goal is to relieve symptoms and reduce inflammation. Antidiarrheal and anti-inflammatory drugs as well as corticosteroids may be prescribed. Proper nutrition and the use of nutritional supplements may also be indicated. Crohn's disease often requires surgery when the intestine is obstructed or for lesions that do not heal with other therapies.

GASTROESOPHAGEAL REFLUX DISEASE

☐ Also known as: GERD

☐ Description: A chronic condition caused by backflow of stomach acids into the esophagus due to a defect or malfunction of the esophageal sphincter, resulting in inflammation and pain. Symptoms often present following ingestion of certain foods, medications, drugs, caffeine, or alcohol.

☐ Causes

o Alcohol consumption

o Caffeinated drinks

o Carbonated drinks

o Chocolate

o Fatty foods

o Medications (such as antihistamines and antidepressants)

o Tobacco products

o Weight gain

☐ Clinical presentation

o Chest/epigastric pain

o Dark or bloody stool

o Esophageal ulcers

- o Esophagitis

- o Excessive salvation

- o Reflux (heartburn)

- o Sensation of a lump in the throat or chest

- o Shortness of breath

- o Sinusitis

- o Sore throat

- □ Management: The most common treatment techniques include avoiding meals late in the evening or prior to lying down, elevating the head while supine or sleeping (to reduce reflux), and avoidance of food and drink that triggers reflux. Cessation of smoking and alcohol use can also aid in the relief of symptoms. Medications that promote tightening of the esophageal sphincter may be prescribed. Antacids may also be effective. Surgery may be an option when other conservative therapies fail.

ULCERATIVE COLITIS

- □ Description: An inflammatory bowel disease characterized by the chronic inflammation and ulceration of the intestinal mucosa, most commonly involving the distal colon, rectum, and anus. The condition can affect persons of any age, but usually occurs in people between the ages of 15 and 30 and between the ages of 50 and 70.

- □ Causes: Ulcerative colitis is idiopathic in nature

- □ Clinical presentation

  - o Abdominal cramping

  - o Anemia or hypovolemia

  - o Anorexia

  - o Arthralgia

  - o Bloody stool

  - o Diarrhea

  - o Fatigue

- o Impaired growth (in children)

- o Intermittent fever

- o Rebound tenderness

- o Skin lesions

- o Urgency to defecate

- o Voluntary or involuntary guarding of the abdominals

- o Watery stools with mucus and pus

- o Weight loss

- □ Management: Most patients with ulcerative colitis can be treated on an outpatient basis. Patients may be prescribed anti-inflammatory medications as well as corticosteroids (oral or IV) and immunomodulating agents. The use of probiotics may also aid in relieving symptoms. Diet should avoid uncooked vegetables, seeds, nuts, and high roughage. In severe cases, surgical removal of the colon may be indicated.

RENAL, UROGENITAL, AND REPRODUCTIVE SYSTEMS

- □ Cystitis

- □ Ectopic pregnancy

- □ Endometriosis

- □ Pelvic inflammatory disease

- □ Human papillomavirus

- □ Hydrocele

- □ Ovarian cyst

- □ Nephrolithiasis

- □ Premenstrual syndrome

- □ Prostatitis

- □ Pyelonephritis

- □ Uterine fibroids

- □ Toxic shock syndrome

- □ Vaginitis

- □ Varicocele

Rehberg RS, Rehberg JS.
Cram Session in General Medical Conditions:
A Handbook for Students & Clinicians (pp. 103-118).
© 2012 Taylor & Francis Group.

CYSTITIS

- □ Also known as: Bladder infection

- □ Description: Bladder inflammation, usually secondary to urinary tract infection.

- □ Causes

  - o Infection

  - o Obstruction of urinary flow (such as by a kidney stone)

  - o Prolapsed uterus or bladder or other structural defect

- □ Clinical presentation

  - o Frequent urination

  - o Pain during urination

  - o Pain in the perineum

  - o Urinary urgency

- □ Management: Antibiotics are effective in treating cystitis caused by infection. Other treatment options may be necessary if the condition is a result of structural defect or obstruction.

ECTOPIC PREGNANCY

- □ Also known as: Tubal pregnancy

- □ Description: An abnormal pregnancy in which a fertilized egg implantation occurs outside of the uterus, most commonly in one of the fallopian tubes. Ectopic pregnancy is the leading cause of pregnancy-related death (occurring in 1 of 150 pregnancies). Chances of ectopic pregnancy increase if the mother has a history of previous tubal disease, ectopic pregnancy, or induced abortion.

- □ Causes

  - o Conception after tubal ligation

  - o Pelvic inflammatory disease

  - o History of prior ectopic pregnancy

  - o History of tubal surgery

- o Increasing age

- o Ruptured appendix

- o Smoking

- o "T-shaped" uterus

- □ Clinical presentation

  - o Abdominal pain

  - o Pelvic pain

  - o Amenorrhea

  - o Endometriosis

  - o Vaginal bleeding

  - o Breast fullness

  - o Cramping

  - o Dyspareunia

  - o Fatigue

  - o Nausea

- □ Management: Diagnosis can be confirmed with a positive urine pregnancy test. Blood test (hCG) and ultrasound can determine how far along the pregnancy is. Ectopic pregnancies cannot become a normal pregnancy. Recent management involves the medication methotrexate, which ends the pregnancy. If the pregnancy is a few weeks along, surgery is required, with every attempt made to save the fallopian tube.

- □ Additional information: A ruptured ectopic pregnancy is a medical emergency because rupture can lead to shock and severe hemorrhage.

ENDOMETRIOSIS

- □ Description: Endometriosis is the presence of endometrial glands and stroma outside of the uterus. Endometrial tissue may be present on the ovaries, bowels, bladder, or behind the uterus, and in rare instances may grow in other parts of the body. Endometriosis occurs in about 10% of women in the United States.

- Causes: The etiology of endometriosis is still relatively unknown. However, there are several theories as to the cause, including endometrial cell migration during fetal development and the expulsion of cells to the peritoneal cavity during menstruation.

- Clinical presentation

  o Asymptomatic

  o Extreme abdominal pain either a few days before the menstrual cycle begins or during the first few days of flow

  o Back pain

  o Dysmenorrheal

  o Heavy menstrual bleeding

  o Low back pain during menses

  o Pelvic pain

  o Premenstrual dyspareunia

- Management: The diagnosis of endometriosis is often made based on clinical presentation and/or inability to get pregnant. It can be confirmed with a diagnostic laparoscopy to directly visualize the reproductive organs for endometrial tissue.

Pain can be treated with ibuprofen or naprosyn. Hormone treatment can reduce endometrial tissue growth. These medications include oral contraceptives, progesterone, Danazol, and gonadotropin-releasing hormone agonists. Surgical intervention may be required to remove endometrial cells and resulting scar tissue. Unfortunately, drugs are not successful in treating the infertility caused by endometriosis.

PELVIC INFLAMMATORY DISEASE

- Also known as: PID

- Description: An infectious and inflammatory disorder of the female reproductive tract. Infection spreads from the cervix into the uterus and fallopian tubes. PID may result in scarring of the fallopian tubes and pelvis, leading to infertility.

- Risk factors

  o Women who have been menstruating for less than 25 years

- o Living in an area with a high prevalence of STDs

- o First intercourse at a young age

- o Multiple sexual partners

- o Inconsistent or no contraception

- o Delayed treatment of infection

- □ Causes: The most common causes of PID are *Chlamydia trachomatis* and *Neisseria gonorrhoeae*. *Escherichia coli* is also known to cause PID.

- □ Clinical presentation

  - o Pelvic and/or lower abdominal pain, usually just prior to or just after the start of menstrual cycle

  - o Involuntary guarding

  - o Laboratory documentation of cervical infection with *C trachomatis* or *N gonorrhoeae*

  - o Rebound tenderness

  - o Uterine tenderness

  - o Abnormal vaginal discharge

  - o Dysuria

  - o Fever

  - o Chills

  - o Nausea

  - o Vomiting

- □ Management: Early treatment of PID is antibiotic therapy. Abscesses in the pelvic and fallopian tubes, if present, must be drained. Previous sexual partners must be examined to reduce risk of STDs and—if positive—must be treated as well.

HUMAN PAPILLOMAVIRUS

- □ Description: Human papillomavirus (HPV) is the most common sexually transmitted infection in the United States. In most cases, infection does not produce symptoms; however, genital warts may be produced in both males and females. Persistent infection may pre-dispose infected individuals to malignancies such as cervical, penile, anal, and vulvar cancers.

□ Causes: HPV is transmitted through sexual contact, most commonly during vaginal and anal sex, but can also be transmitted via genital to genital contact. In rare cases, transmission of the virus from an infected pregnant mother to the child is possible during childbirth.

□ Clinical presentation: A pelvic exam with the papanicolaou test (PAP smear) is often required to detect cervical infection in women. Genital warts usually present in clusters or large masses. Lesions will appear flat and white.

□ Management: The best and most effective treatment of HPV is preven-tion. Routine PAP tests are recommended for women because cervical cancer can be treated if diagnosed in the early stages. An HPV vac-cine is available to protect both males and females from HPV. Genital warts produced by HPV can be removed using medication.

HYDROCELE

□ Description: A collection of fluid in the tunica vaginalis testis in males; this can also occur in females along the canal of Nuck. They are common in newborns. Injury, surgery, inflammation, infection, and cancer can lead to hydroceles in individuals older than 40 years.

□ Causes: The cause of a hydrocele is usually unknown.

□ Clinical presentation

    o Asymptomatic

    o Nontender fullness

    o Swelling and redness surrounding the testes

□ Management: Most hydroceles do not need treatment. Larger hydro-celes may be surgically removed.

OVARIAN CYST

□ Description: A fluid-filled sac that forms inside or arises from an ovary. Ovarian cysts are most common in women from puberty to menopause. Cysts may be asymptomatic but can cause pain if the cyst ruptures or impinges on other organs.

- ☐ Causes: There are no known risk factors for ovarian cysts.

- ☐ Clinical presentation

  - ○ Most women are asymptomatic

  - ○ Abdominal or pelvic pain

  - ○ Abdominal tenderness

  - ○ Pain with intercourse

  - ○ Pain during bowel movements

  - ○ Fever

- ☐ Management: CT scan, ultrasound, MRI, or pelvic exam may be used to confirm diagnosis in symptomatic patients. Patients with simple cysts who are asymptomatic do not require treatment. Patients with persistent cysts that are 5 to 10 cm and are symptomatic may require surgical removal of the cyst.

NEPHROLITHIASIS

- ☐ Also known as: Urinary stones, kidney stones, urinary calculi

- ☐ Description: The presence of calculi (stones) in the kidney or ureters. Calculi can vary in size, ranging from microscopic to several centimeters in diameter. Almost 80% of calculi are made of calcium.

- ☐ Causes

  - ○ Hyperthyroidism

  - ○ High-protein diet

  - ○ Low magnesium levels

  - ○ Hypercalciuria

  - ○ Low fluid intake

  - ○ Family history

- ☐ Clinical presentation

  - ○ Abdominal distention

  - ○ Chills

- o Fever

- o Hematuria

- o Increased urination

- o Nausea

- o Severe, intermittent pain

- o Vomiting

- □ Management: Calculi that do not cause symptoms or complications do not need treatment. Consumption of large amounts of fluid may aid in passing the calculi through the urinary tract. Pain medication may be used to manage discomfort associated with the condition. Depending on the size of the calculi, surgery may be indicated for patients who are experiencing extreme pain, obstruction, or infection.

PREMENSTRUAL SYNDROME

- □ Also known as: PMS

- □ Description: A group of physical, psychological, behavioral, and emotional symptoms that usually present 7 to 10 days prior to onset of menstruation. Symptoms can often disrupt normal daily activity. Often subsides with onset of menstrual flow.

- □ Causes: There is no true cause of PMS. The following several conditions are considered possible factors:

  - o Serotonin deficiency

  - o Magnesium deficiency

  - o Calcium deficiency

  - o Exaggerated response to normal hormone changes

  - o Increased release of endorphins

- □ Clinical presentation

  - o Agitation

  - o Anger

  - o Insomnia

  - o Irritability

o Lethargy

o Water retention

o Weight gain

□ Management: Exercise, medication, and behavioral modification are commonly used methods of managing the effects of PMS. Premenstrual dysphoric disorder (PMDD)—which is characterized by severe depression, irritability, or tension before menstruation—may require medication or surgical intervention.

PROSTATITIS

□ Also known as: Acute bacterial prostatitis, chronic bacterial prostatitis, chronic nonbacterial prostatitis

□ Description: Inflammation or infection of the prostate. Chronic nonbacterial prostatitis accounts for 90% of cases. Acute bacterial prostatitis is the least common but presents with the most severe symptoms.

□ Risk factors

o Recurrent bacterial infections of the prostate

o Prostatic calculi

o History of a medical procedure involving an instrument inserted into the bladder

o Enlarged prostate

o Rectal intercourse

□ Clinical presentation

o Burning

o Chills

o Dysuria

o Fever

o Hematuria

o Increased urinary frequency and/or urgency

- o Lower back pain

- o Perineal pain

- o Voiding dysfunction

- □ Management: The most common management for prostatitis is oral or intravenous antibiotic treatment, depending on the type of infection. Anti-inflammatory medications, pain medications, muscle relaxants, and stool softeners can often aid in relieving symptoms. Surgery is reserved for severe cases.

PYELONEPHRITIS

- □ Also known as: Kidney infection

- □ Description: A bacterial kidney infection usually resulting from bacteria spread from the bladder. The most common bacteria causing this condition is *E coli.*

- □ Causes

  - o Bladder infection

  - o Urinary tract surgery

  - o Insertion of objects into the bladder and/or urethra (eg, catheter, cystoscope)

  - o Prostatitis

  - o Kidney stones

  - o Urinary tract defects that impede normal flow of urine

- □ Clinical presentation

  - o Fever

  - o Frequent and/or urgent urination

  - o Hematuria

  - o Nausea

  - o Pain and/or burning during urination

  - o Pain in the back, flank, and/or groin

  - o Vomiting

- Management: Urinalysis is used to confirm the diagnosis and presence of bacteria. Antibiotic medication is effective in treating the bacterial infection. Severe cases may require hospitalization. Surgery may be required for anatomic abnormalities.

UTERINE FIBROIDS

- Also known as: Uterine leiomyoma

- Description: A benign tumor of the smooth muscle of the uterus that can appear during the reproductive years. Uterine fibroids are the most common noncancerous tumor in women of childbearing age, occurring in approximately 25% of all women.

- Cause: Uterine fibroids are idiopathic in nature; however, risk factors include obesity and race. African-American women are at highest risk.

- Clinical presentation
  - Abdominal distention
  - Abnormal uterine bleeding
  - Constipation
  - Edema
  - Genitourinary dysfunction
  - Infertility
  - Intestinal obstruction
  - Pelvic pain and/or pressure

- Management: Surgical removal of uterine fibroids may be necessary. Hormone therapy, gonadotrophin-releasing hormones (GnRH), or selective estrogen receptor modulators (SERMs) may be used to shrink fibroids. Fibroid embolization is a procedure that can also shrink fibroids. Myomectomy will remove the fibroid; hysterectomy removes the entire uterus.

TOXIC SHOCK SYNDROME

- Description: A collection of severe, rapid onset symptoms caused by infection from *Staphylococcus aureus* or group *A streptococci*. Symptoms include fever, hypotension, rash, and organ failure.

- Causes: Toxic shock syndrome is most commonly associated with menstruating women and the misuse of vaginal tampons. Infection may also occur following surgery.

- Clinical presentation

  - Fever

  - Hypotension

  - Full body skin rash resembling sunburn

  - Multiple organ failure

  - Chills

  - Confusion

  - Diarrhea

  - Edema

  - Muscle aches

  - Sore throat

  - Renal dysfunction

  - Vomiting

- Management: Diagnosis is based upon symptoms, history, and physical exam and is confirmed through blood culture. Immediate medical care and hospitalization is indicated. Removal of any foreign objects (such as tampons and diaphragms) is required. Surgical wounds or areas where bacteria can accumulate should be irrigated.

VAGINITIS

- Also known as: Vulvovaginitis

- Description: Infection or inflammation of the vagina; vulvovaginits affects the vulva and vagina. It is the most common gynecological condition seen in women of childbearing age. Susceptibility for infection increases when vaginal pH is disturbed. Feminine hygiene products, antibiotics, sexually transmitted diseases, sexual intercourse, and stress are all factors that can affect vaginal pH.

- Risk factors
  - Recent antibiotic use
  - Uncontrolled diabetes
  - Pregnancy
    - Birth control pills
    - Endocrine disorders
    - Corticosteroids
- Causes
  - Bacteria
  - Trichomonas vaginalis (sexually transmitted)
  - Chlamydia (sexually transmitted)
  - Yeast; Candida
  - Viruses, including HPV and herpes simplex virus (HSV)
  - Noninfectious
    - Foreign bodies
      - Fistulas
      - Radiation
      - Tumors of the genital tract
- Clinical presentation
  - Bacterial
    - White or discolored "fishy" smelling discharge
    - Painful urination
    - Irritation of vulva and vagina
  - Yeast
    - Thick, white, "cottage cheese" discharge
    - Irritation of vulva and vagina

- o Trichomonas
  - Frothy, green-yellow, foul smelling discharge
  - Burning with urination
  - Irritation of vulva and vagina
  - Dyspareunia
  - Lower abdominal pain
- o Chlamydia
  - Asymptomatic
  - Discharge may or may not be present
  - Light bleeding after intercourse
  - Abdominal and pelvic pain
- o Viruses
  - Painful lesions
  - Genital warts
- o Noninfectious
  - Itching
  - Dyspareunia
  - Vaginal dryness
- □ Management: Treatment is specific to the causative agent. Yeast infections are treated with antifungals in either pill form or suppository. Bacterial infections are treated with clindamycin or metronidazole. Chlamydial infections are treated with azithromycin or doxycycline. Trichomonal infections are treated with antiprotozoal medications such as metronidazole or tinidazole. Antiviral medications do not cure HSV or HPV; they help the lesions heal faster. In noninfectious vaginitis, the probable cause should be addressed.

VARICOCELE

- Description: Dilation of the venous plexus of the scrotum (usually the left) due to a valvular defect of the scrotal veins. This condition occurs in about 10% to 20% of the male population and is believed to interfere with testicular thermoregulation.

- Causes: A defect in the valves of the affected veins.

- Clinical presentation

  - Dull ache on the affected side and a long spermatic cord

  - On palpation, affected vessels feel full, and are reminiscent of a bundle of worms

  - Scrotal pain/heaviness

  - Symptoms often present when standing upright and resolve upon assuming a supine position

- Management: Most varicoceles are asymptomatic and do not require treatment. Surgery may be indicated in patients who experience pain or those who are infertile.

8

EAR, NOSE, AND THROAT CONDITIONS

- ☐ Sinusitis

- ☐ Allergic rhinitis

- ☐ Benign paroxysmal positional vertigo

- ☐ Labyrinthitis

- ☐ Otitis externa

- ☐ Otitis media

- ☐ Ruptured tympanic membrane

- ☐ Tinnitus

- ☐ Tonsillitis

Rehberg RS, Rehberg JS.
*Cram Session in General Medical Conditions:
A Handbook for Students & Clinicians* (pp. 119-126).
© 2012 Taylor & Francis Group.

SINUSITIS

☐ Also known as: Acute sinusitis, chronic sinusitis, chronic hyperplastic sinusitis

☐ Description: An inflammation of the sinuses. Sinusitis can be classified as acute sinusitis, with symptoms lasting between 2 and 8 weeks or chronic sinusitis, with symptoms lasting longer than 8 weeks. Chronic hyperplastic sinusitis is a form of chronic sinusitis characterized by polyps present in the sinuses and nose.

☐ Causes: Sinusitis can be caused by allergy, inhaled pollutants, or by bacterial, fungal, or viral infection. Sinusitis may be preceded by a cold.

☐ Clinical presentation

  o Congestion

  o Cough

  o Fatigue

  o Fever

  o Headache

  o Postnasal drip

  o Weakness

☐ Management: Nasal decongestants, analgesics, and the use of saline spray and vaporizers are common methods of treatment. In some acute cases, antibiotics may be prescribed. Chronic sinusitis may require surgery to improve drainage and reduce nasal passage blockage. Chronic hyperplastic sinusitis may require the removal of sinus and nasal polyps.

ALLERGIC RHINITIS

☐ Also known as: Hay fever, pollinosis

☐ Description: Inflammation of the nasal mucosa due to allergic reaction. Often referred to as hay fever.

☐ Causes: Environmental triggers such as pollen, grass, and ragweed can cause this condition, with the severity often dependent upon the concentration of the allergen in the air and weather conditions (warmer, dry, and windy days). Animal dander, dust, and mold are other common causes.

- Clinical presentation: The most common symptoms include one or more of the following:

  - Difficulty breathing through the nose (nasal congestion)

  - Impaired sense of smell

  - Itching of the eyes, nose, mouth, or throat

  - Lacrimation

  - Nasal discharge

  - Postnasal drip

  - Sore throat

  - Sneezing

  - Suborbital swelling

- Management: The best method of treatment involves prevention through avoidance of triggers. Mild cases of allergic rhinitis may be alleviated with a nasal flush using saline. Oral antihistamines, oral and nasal decongestants, and nasal corticosteroids are effective therapies used for treating symptoms. In cases where allergens cannot be avoided and symptoms persist, immunotherapy may be indicated.

BENIGN PAROXYSMAL POSITIONAL VERTIGO

- Also known as: BPPV, canalithiasis

- Description: An inner ear (labyrinth) disorder characterized by mild to severe short-term vertigo associated with changes in head position

- Causes: Most commonly idiopathic in nature, BPPV can also be caused by trauma and infection. Vertigo is caused when there are rapid changes in head position, such as tipping the head up or down or rising from a supine position. Vertigo is caused by otolith crystals from the vestibule of the inner ear to the semicircular canals.

- Clinical presentation: Sudden change in head position causes one or more of the following:
  - Dizziness
  - Blurred vision
  - Lightheadedness
  - Loss of balance
  - Nausea
  - Nystagmus
  - Unsteadiness
  - Vomiting (in rare cases)
- Management: Canalith repositioning, also known as particle-repositioning or the Epley maneuver, which involves slow maneuvers of head positioning designed to move otolith crystals out of the semicircular canals, may aid in eliminating symptoms. Medication may be prescribed to treat nausea and dizziness. In more severe cases, surgery may be indicated.

LABYRINTHITIS

- Also known as: Meniere's disease, otitis interna, otitis labyrinthica
- Description: Irritation and inflammation of the inner ear, usually following ear or upper respiratory infection
- Causes: Risk factors for labyrinthitis include excessive alcohol consumption, history of allergy, recent ear or respiratory infection, viral illness, smoking, stress, and use of specific medications.
- Clinical presentation: Individuals with labyrinthitis may experience one or more of the following symptoms:
  - Hearing loss
  - Loss of balance
  - Nausea
  - Nystagmus

- o Tinnitus

- o Vertigo

- o Vomiting

- ☐ Management: Acute attacks are best treated with bed rest. Use of antihistamines and sedatives may be used to treat symptoms. Surgical treatment is considered a last resort.

OTITIS EXTERNA

- ☐ Also known as: External otitis, outer ear infection, swimmer's ear

- ☐ Description: An infection of the aural canal

- ☐ Causes: Infection is usually caused by bacteria, which is the most common, or fungi. Chemical irritation such as cosmetics, sprays, or dyes can also cause infection. The condition is common in swimmers and is often called swimmer's ear. Those affected by allergies, eczema, psoriasis, or scalp dermatitis are at increased risk for the condition.

- ☐ Clinical presentation: Symptoms may include itching and pain in the ear, discharge from an infected ear that is usually odorous and white or yellow in color, and swelling of the aural canal.

- ☐ Management: Treatment first involves removal of the infected material from the canal. Vinegar can be applied via ear drops to the canal to aid in restoring acidity in the canal. Corticosteroid drops may also be applied to aid in inflammation. In moderate to severe infections, antibiotic drops may be indicated. Analgesic medication, such as acetaminophen, may be prescribed for pain.

OTITIS MEDIA

- ☐ Also known as: Acute otitis media, chronic otitis media, secretory otitis media

- ☐ Description: An infection of the middle ear, classified as acute, chronic, or secretory

- ☐ Causes: Acute otitis media is caused by a bacterial or viral infection. Risk factors include age (under 2 years), exposure to respiratory infection, secondhand smoke, and allergies. Chronic otitis media is an infection caused by eardrum perforation or chloasma. Secretory otitis media is an accumulation of fluid in the middle ear, most commonly caused by a blockage in the eustachian tube.

- Clinical presentation
  - Discharge from the aural canal
  - Fever
  - Headache
  - Hearing loss
  - History of recent upper respiratory infection
  - Irritability
  - Lethargy
  - Pain in the ear
  - Sensation of fullness in the ear
- Management: Acute otitis media can be treated with acetaminophen or nonsteroidal anti-inflammatory drugs (NSAIDs) for pain relief. Antibiotics may also be prescribed. In severe cases, a myringotomy (a surgical opening made in the tympanic membrane to allow drainage of fluid) may be performed. Treatment of chronic otitis media consists of cleaning of the ear canal, application of acetic acid, hydrocortisone, or antibiotic medication to the ear canal (ear drops). Treatment of secretory otitis media is similar to acute. Patients may also force air past the blockage in the eustachian tube by attempting to exhale with the mouth shut and the nose pinched.

RUPTURED TYMPANIC MEMBRANE

- Also known as: Eardrum perforation
- Description: A hole in the tympanic membrane (eardrum)
- Causes: Otitis media is the most common cause of ruptured tympanic membrane. Other causes include sudden change in atmospheric pressure (explosion, slap to the ear, underwater diving, change in altitude) or damage by a foreign object (such as a cotton swab).
- Clinical presentation
  - Sudden, severe ear pain
  - Bleeding from the ear (possible)
  - Drainage of pus from the ear (possible)

- o Hearing loss

- o Tinnitus

- o Vertigo

- ▫ Management: Diagnosis is confirmed by visual inspection using an otoscope. Ruptures typically heal without treatment. However, antibiotics may be prescribed if infection is present. Ruptures that do not heal within 2 months require surgical repair.

- ▫ Additional information: Persistent hearing loss following perforation may indicate a disruption of the ossicles, which may require surgical repair.

TINNITUS

- ▫ Also known as: Ringing in the ear

- ▫ Description: Noise (ringing, buzzing, or hissing) originating in the ear. Tinnitus is not a disease but a symptom caused by several other conditions.

- ▫ Causes: Most common causes include otitis media, labyrinthitis, impacted cerumen, ruptured tympanic membrane, loud noises, explosions, or a reaction to certain medications.

- ▫ Clinical presentation: Subjective noise experienced by patients and characterized as ringing, buzzing, or hissing. Noise may be more pronounced in quiet environments. Tolerance level of symptoms varies.

- ▫ Management: Primary treatment involves identifying the cause of the symptom. Use of background noise or music may aid in tolerating the symptom. For chronic, long lasting, or severe cases of tinnitus, hearing aids or cochlear implants may aid in reducing the symptom.

TONSILLITIS

- ▫ Also known as: Acute tonsillitis, follicular tonsillitis, acute parenchymatous tonsillitis

- ▫ Description: Inflammation of the tonsils, which is the lymphoid tissue located on either side of the posterior aspect of the throat

- ▫ Causes: The most common cause of tonsillitis is viral infection. Streptococcal infection is also a common cause.

☐ Clinical presentation: Throat pain, especially when swallowing, is the hallmark symptom of tonsillitis. Cough, fever, rhinorrhea, and diarrhea are common in viral infections. Fever, headache, nausea, vomiting, and swollen cervical lymph nodes are common in streptococcal infection. Upon visual inspection, tonsils appear enlarged and red. Presence of exudate is common.

☐ Management: Treatment for tonsillitis primarily consists of symptom management. A throat culture is used to confirm the diagnosis of infection. Antibiotics may be used to treat bacterial infection. Untreated streptococcal infection (eg, strep throat) can lead to rheumatic fever and heart valve damage. Chronic tonsillitis is commonly treated through surgical removal of the tonsils.

INFECTIOUS DISEASE

- □ Acquired immune deficiency syndrome
- □ Varicella-Zoster virus
- □ Herpes simplex
- □ Hand, foot, and mouth disease
- □ Infectious mononucleosis
- □ Lyme disease
- □ Malaria
- □ Measles
- □ Mumps
- □ Rubella
- □ Meningitis
- □ Rabies
- □ Tetanus
- □ Pertussis
- □ Erythema infectiosum

Rehberg RS, Rehberg JS.
Cram Session in General Medical Conditions:
A Handbook for Students & Clinicians (pp. 127-142).
© 2012 Taylor & Francis Group.

ACQUIRED IMMUNODEFICIENCY SYNDROME

□ Description: Infection with human retrovirus known as human immunodeficiency virus (HIV or HIV-1). Following infection with HIV virus, the virus infects CD4+ helper T lymphocytes; as the infection progresses, these CD4+ cells are depleted, leading to immunosuppression. Immunosuppression increases the risk of opportunistic infections. AIDS is the development of one or more opportunistic infections and unusual neoplasms for which there is no other explanation in the presence of evidence of HIV infection. The HIV virus is transmitted via sexual intercourse (vaginal and anal) with an infected individual, parenteral contact with infected blood or blood products, and maternal-fetal spread.

□ Diagnosis: Sequential testing for the detection of anti-HIV antibodies using the enzyme-linked immunosorbent assay (ELISA) test. If testing is positive, Western blot is used to confirm the diagnosis. Antibodies usually develop within 3 months of exposure. Rapid tests are available for HIV infection, but should be followed with confirmatory testing.

□ Manifestations

  o Centers for Disease Control and Prevention (CDC) classification of clinical syndromes:

  ■ Group I: Acute seroconversion illness

    • Mononucleosis-like infection; supportive treatment. Encephalopathy, meningitis, myelopathy, and neuropathy can also occur.

  ■ Group II: Asymptomatic infection

    • The length of time between exposure and the development of disease is, on average, 10 years. CD4 counts begin to fall during this time.

  ■ Group III: Persistent generalized adenopathy

    • Nodes measure > 1 cm in diameter at 2 or more extrainguinal sites that persist for longer than 3 months with no other explanation than HIV.

- Group IV: Other disease; includes acquired immunodeficiency syndrome (AIDS) with a CD4 lymphocyte count below 200 cells/mL

  - Subgroup A—Constitutional disease: Fever, weight loss, diarrhea

  - Subgroup B—Neurologic disease: HIV encephalopathy is most common

  - Subgroup C—Secondary infectious diseases: *Pneumocystis carinii* pneumonia, *Candida albicans* (oral thrush, esophagitis), cytomegalovirus (colitis, retinitis, pneumonitis), *M tuberculosis*, *Toxoplasma gondii* (brain abscesses), *Cryptococcus neoformans* (meningitis), *Cryptosporidium* (chronic diarrhea), *Mycobacterium avium* complex

  - Subgroup D—Secondary neoplasms: Kaposi's sarcoma, lymphomas

  - Subgroup E—Other conditions

  - Management: Prevention through education and counseling on safe sex; encouragement of IV drug abusers not to share needles; and avoidance of breast feeding. Health care workers should practice universal precautions.

□ Treatment: Antiretroviral therapy, chemoprophylaxis for opportunistic infections (specific for each pathogen), and treatment of opportunistic infections and neoplasms (specific for each infection).

  o Post-needle stick: Thorough washing, encourage bleeding; post-exposure prophylaxis can reduce the risk of transmission following exposure. Testing is done at 6 weeks, 12 weeks, and 6 months post-exposure.

VARICELLA-ZOSTER VIRUS

□ Also known as: Varicella or chickenpox, Herpes zoster or shingles

□ Description: A highly contagious member of the herpes virus family. Primary infection results in chickenpox. The virus lays dormant in the dorsal root ganglia. Reactivation results in shingles. Transmission of the virus occurs via direct contact with vesicular fluid from an infected individual or from respiratory secretions. Individuals are contagious from 1 to 2 days before onset of rash to crusting of all lesions. The incubation period is usually 14 to 16 days, ranges from 10 to 21 days. Varicella is more severe in adults than in young children. Triggering factors for shingles are immunosuppression, trauma, stress, and increasing age.

- □ Clinical presentation
  - o Chickenpox
    - ■ Fever
    - ■ Malaise
    - ■ Generalized pruritic rash that has varying stages: papules-vesicles ("dew drop on a petal") and pustules crusting resolution
    - ■ Complications of chickenpox
      - • Bacterial superinfection of the skin
      - • Central nervous system (CNS) involvement
      - • Pneumonia
  - o Shingles
    - ■ Begins with approximately 5 days of radicular pain
    - ■ Vesicular rash follows presenting with a unilateral distribution in multiple, contiguous dermatomes
    - ■ Postherpetic neuralgia, or pain that persists despite resolution of the rash, can exist for weeks to months.
- □ Diagnosis: Usually made clinically. Tzanck smears of vesicle base scrapings have been used.
- □ Management
  - o Chickenpox: Treatment is symptomatic. Oral acyclovir is recommended for individuals at risk for severe cases and should be administered within 72 hours from onset of rash. IV acyclovir is recommended for immunocompromised patients. Antipruritics can be administered. Care should be taken to prevent secondary skin infections. Salicylates or salicylate-containing products should not be administered to children due to the increased risk of Reye syndrome.

- Shingles: Oral famciclovir, valacyclovir, or acyclovir. IV acyclovir is indicated for the immcompromised patient. Analgesics can be given for acute neuritis or postherpetic neuritis. Care should be taken to prevent secondary skin infections.

- Immunizations for varicella and herpes zoster are available.

HERPES SIMPLEX

- Also known as: Cold sores/herpes labialis; genital herpes

- Description: Skin lesions of the perioral and anogenital surfaces caused by herpes simplex virus Types 1 and 2. Type 1 most commonly causes orofacial lesions. Type 2 commonly causes genital herpes, although Type 1 can also cause genital lesions. Asymptomatic viral shedding accounts for the most common mode of transmission. The virus can also be transmitted through direct contact with active lesions, contaminated saliva, or by sexual contact. Reactivation of the virus occurs following illness, fever, stress, exposure to sunlight, immune suppression, fatigue, menses, or skin abrasion.

- Diagnosis: Available testing includes direct immunofluorescence of vesicle base scrapings, viral culture, serologic testing for HSV antibodies, and Tzanck smear.

- Clinical presentation

  - Lesions may be preceded by tingling, burning, and pain

  - Lesions appear as grouped or clustered vesicles and erosions on an erythematous base

  - Swollen and tender lymph nodes may be present

  - Lesions typically heal in approximately 7 to 10 days

- Management: Prevention of lesions with prophylactic oral antivirals. Sunscreen can prevent sun-induced lesions. Treatment of active lesions includes oral and topical antiviral agents.

HAND, FOOT, AND MOUTH DISEASE

- Also known as: Coxsackievirus

- Description: A self-limiting illness. A highly contagious illness spread by oral-to-oral or fecal-to-oral route.

- Diagnosis: Diagnosis can be made via isolation of the virus from throat washings.

- Clinical presentation

  o Small vesicles on the fingers, palms, and soles that often resemble red halos

  o Ulcerations on the tongue; oral mucosa may appear

  o Illness may include prodrome of fever, malaise, and upper respiratory symptoms

- Management: Treatment is supportive. Topical lidocaine can be used for oral ulcerations.

INFECTIOUS MONONUCLEOSIS

- Also known as: Mono

- Description: Epstein-Barr virus is the most common cause of mononucleosis. It is transmitted via oral secretions. The incubation period is typically 30 to 50 days.

- Diagnosis: Complete blood count shows elevated white count with atypical lymphocytosis. Monospot tests are more sensitive than heterophile tests but can be negative during the first week of symptoms.

- Clinical presentation

  o Fever

  o Headache

  o Myalgias

  o Nausea

  o Anorexia

  o Sore throat

  o Pharyngitis can be severe, often with exudative tonsillitis

  o Generalized lymphadenopathy

  o Hepatosplenomegaly

  o Pruritic rash almost always occurs in individuals treated with ampicillin or amoxicillin

- o Initial symptoms can last 1 to 3 weeks; malaise can persist for months

- □ Management: Treatment is symptomatic. Contact sports should be avoided until the spleen is no longer palpable to avoid splenic rupture; typically 4 to 6 weeks. Steroids can be used for severe cases.

LYME DISEASE

- □ Description: A bacterial illness transmitted from the bite of a tick infected with *Borrelia burgdorferi*. It is the most common tick-borne illness in the United States.

- □ Diagnosis: Erythema migrans (EM) is indicative of Lyme disease and treatment should begin immediately. Laboratory testing, as recommended by the CDC, is a 2-step process: Lyme titer and Western blot are necessary to confirm a positive titer.

- □ Clinical presentation: There are 3 stages of Lyme disease. Progression of the disease occurs if proper treatment is not received.

  - o Early localized stage: Manifests as an erythematous rash at or near the site of the tick bite. The disease is characterized by an enlarging rash or a central spot with rings (bull's eye). The incubation period from the bite to the appearance of a rash ranges from 1 to 55 days, median 11 days. Systemic symptoms include fever, fatigue, malaise, arthralgias, headache, and neck pain.

  - o Early disseminated stage: Occurs within days of the onset of EM. Secondary annular lesions, smaller than the primary lesion, develop. Neurologic manifestations such as cranial nerve palsies, peripheral neuropathies, and meningitis occur. Cardiac involvement is less common and includes conduction abnormalities, arrhythmias, and myopericarditis. Severe fatigue, migratory musculoskeletal pain, and headache are common.

  - o Late stage: Occurs within 1 year after onset of illness. Polyarthritis in large joints, especially in the knees, develops. CNS manifestations include confusion, disorientation, and dizziness.

- □ Management: Initial treatment within 72 hours of tick removal is a single dose of doxycycline. In early disease, preferred treatment is doxycycline. Penicillin (alternative is cefuroxime) is recommended for children under the age of 8 and others in whom treatment with a tetracycline is contraindicated (such as in pregnant or lactating women).

Treatment is for 21 days. In later stages, doxycycline, ceftriaxone, and high-dose penicillin can be used.

MALARIA

☐ Description: Malaria is caused by protozoa of the genus *Plasmodium*. There are 4 species that infect humans: *P falciparum, P vivax, P ovale,* and *P malariae*. It is endemic to most of the tropical and subtropical areas of the world. It is acquired from the bite of a female anopheline mosquito. *P falciparum* malaria is the most severe form of the disease. Once treated, relapse is rare. Non-*P falciparum* malaria is more benign in nature. Relapse can occur due to the persistence of hypnozoites in the liver. Other manifestations include anemia and thrombocytopenia. Hemolysis may lead to jaundice and pallor. Hepatosplenomegaly may be present. Death is usually caused by *P falciparum*.

☐ Diagnosis: Diagnosis of malaria is made with blood smear stained with Giemsa stain.

☐ Clinical presentation: Symptoms may be paroxysmal; if proper treatment is not received, fever and paroxysms can be cyclical

  o High fever and chills

  o Sweats

  o Headache

  o Malaise

  o Myalgias

  o Nausea, vomiting, and diarrhea

☐ Management: Treatment regimens depend on the cause of infection; if unknown or mixed infection, treat as if chloroquine-resistant.

  o *P falciparum*—Should be treated with quinine sulfate and doxycycline; severe infection requires parenteral therapy with quinidine gluconate and doxycycline

  o Non-*P falciparum*—Oral chloroquine should be administered. Relapses should be treated with chloroquine and primaquine.

Prevention can be achieved with appropriate chemoprophylaxis and proper measures to limit mosquito exposure. Protective clothing, such as long-sleeved shirts and pants; mosquito netting (impregnated with insecticide); and repellents containing diethyltoluamide (DEET) should also be used. Chemoprophylaxis should be determined by the regions to be visited and should begin prior to travel and should continue until arrival home, depending on the chemoprophylaxis indicated.

MEASLES

- Also known as: Rubeola

- Description: Highly contagious viral disease caused by a virus in the paramyxovirus family. The virus is transmitted by the airborne spread of infectious droplets. The incubation period is 10 to 15 days from exposure. Individuals are contagious 1 to 2 days prior to onset of symptoms up to 4 days after the rash develops.

- Diagnosis: Confirmation of diagnosis via serological testing

- Clinical presentation: Prodrome of fever, malaise, cough, irritability, coryza (nasal obstruction, sore throat, and sneezing), conjunctivitis, and Koplik's spots

  - Koplik's spots look like tiny grains of salt surrounded by a red ring that typically appear on the buccal mucosa and inner lower lip. They are pathognomonic of measles.

Rash typically appears 4 days later and is composed of erythematous maculopapules that coalesce. It starts on the forehead, spreads downward over the face, neck, trunk, and feet, and resolves in order of appearance. Complications include pneumonia, croup, bronchitis, otitis media, diarrhea, and encephalomyelitis.

- Management: Prevention by vaccination. Treatment is symptomatic.

MUMPS

- Description: Systemic viral illness caused by a virus in the paramyxovirus family that usually produces swelling of the salivary glands, particularly the parotid glands. The virus is transmitted via infected respiratory tract secretions. The incubation period is usually 16 to 18 days. The infected individual is contagious 1 to 2 days prior to the onset of parotid swelling, which lasts 5 days.

- Diagnosis: Confirmed by isolation of the virus in a culture or via serology

- □ Clinical presentation
  - ○ Sudden parotid swelling and tenderness; often bilateral
  - ○ Fever
  - ○ Malaise
  - ○ Headache
  - ○ Other manifestations
    - ▪ Orchitis (pain and swelling of the testicles)
    - ▪ Pancreatitis
    - ▪ Meningitis
    - ▪ Thyroiditis
    - ▪ Myocarditis
    - ▪ Thrombocytopenia
    - ▪ Glomerulonephritis
    - ▪ Arthritis
- □ Management: Prevention with immunization. Treatment is supportive.

RUBELLA

- □ Also known as: German measles
- □ Description: A respiratory illness caused by a member of the *Togavirus* family. It is transmitted via inhalation of respiratory secretions. Incubation period is 14 to 21 days. Illness is contagious from 1 week prior to the development of a rash until 15 days afterward. Rubella occurring in pregnant woman during the first trimester can be passed to the developing fetus and is known as congenital rubella syndrome. Manifestations in the newborn include congenital heart effects, eye lesions, microcephaly, deafness, and mental retardation.
  - ○ Fine, pink maculapapular rash presents initially on forehead, spreading downward over face, trunk, and extremities within 24 hours. It resolves within 3 days.
- □ Diagnosis: Confirmed by serology

- Clinical presentation
  - Prodrome
    - Fever
    - Malaise
    - Anorexia
    - Headache
    - Coryza
    - Palatal erythema
    - Conjunctivitis
    - Lymphadenopathy
    - Transient polyarthralgias and polyarthritis occur in young women
- Management: Prevention with immunization. Treatment is symptomatic.

MENINGITIS

- Description: Inflammation of the meninges due to infection. Meningitis should be considered in any patient with neurologic symptoms and fever and should be considered a medical emergency. Meningitis can be typed as purulent (meningococcal or bacterial), aseptic (typically viral), and granulomatous (mycobacterial, fungal). *Streptococcus pneumoniae* and *Neisseria meningitides* are the most common causes of bacterial meningitis in adults.
- Risk factors
  - Crowding
  - Poverty
  - Malnutrition
  - Head injury
  - Immunosuppression
  - Sinusitis

- o Mastoiditis

- o Pneumonia

- o Alcoholism

- o Diabetes mellitus

- ☐ Diagnosis: Lumbar puncture is standard for diagnosis. Cerebral spinal fluid (CSF) specimen is obtained and sent for testing: gram stain, culture, cell count, glucose, and protein. Head CT scan is performed prior to lumbar tap if elevated intracranial pressure is suspected. It is done to rule out a space-occupying lesion in order to prevent brainstem herniation and death. Blood cultures and blood count should also be performed.

- ☐ Clinical presentation

- o Headache

- o Fever

- o Neck and back stiffness

- o Impaired consciousness

- o Seizures

- o Vomiting

- o Rash

- o Positive Kernig's and Brudzinski's signs

  - ▪ Kernig's sign: Pain in the hamstring with passive extension of the knee with the hip flexed to 90 degrees

  - ▪ Brudzinski's sign: Flexion of the knee in response to flexion of the neck

- ☐ Management: Initial antibacterial therapy (prior to testing) should be administered if bacterial meningitis is suspected. Antimicrobial treatment is specific to the causative organism. Aseptic meningitis is usually self-limiting; treatment is supportive. Bacterial meningitis is contagious, and close contacts should receive prophylactic treatment. Vaccinations for bacterial meningitis are available.

RABIES

- □ Description: An RNA virus of the rhabdovirus group. The virus is typically passed in the infected saliva from the bite of an infected animal. The incubation period is an average of 1 to 2 months, but can be from 5 days to more than 1 year. Infected animals are typically found in the wild and include raccoons, bats, skunks, and foxes; fewer cases occur in domesticated cats and dogs.

- □ Clinical presentation
  - o Acute illness presents with the following nonspecific symptoms:
    - Fever
    - Headache
    - Malaise
    - Nausea and vomiting
    - Anorexia
    - Myalgias
    - Fatigue
    - Sore throat
    - Cough
  - o Symptoms may proceed to the following CNS manifestations:
    - Confusion
    - Muscle spasms
    - Seizures
    - Anxiety
    - Agitation
  - o Paralysis may be exhibited
  - o Median survival within onset of symptoms is 4 days; recovery is rare

- Management: All wounds should be cleaned. Tetanus toxoid and antibiotic should be administered. Further treatment depends on the following several factors:

  o Bite from a domestic animal—Observation for abnormal behavior; if any develops, the brain tissue of the animal should be examined for disease. If the animal remains normal, no further action is needed.

  o Bite from a suspected animal—Capture of the animal and examination of the brain tissue. If the animal is not able to be captured, rabies should be assumed and treatment should begin.

- Treatment

  o Concurrent administration

    - Passive immunoprophylaxis—Human rabies immune globulin (RIG) administered locally at the wound site and intramuscularly.

    - Active immunoprophylaxis—Human rabies vaccine administered intramuscularly on days 0, 3, 7, 14, and 28.

- Additional information: Individuals in high-risk groups can receive pre-exposure immunization given intramuscularly on days 0, 7, 21, or 28. Titers should be checked every 2 to 6 years.

TETANUS

- Also known as: Lockjaw, or generalized tetanus

- Description: A neurologic disease. In a contaminated wound, the bacterium *Clostridium tetani* produces the exotoxin tetanospasmin, which causes muscle spasms and rigidity. Symptoms typically develop within 7 to 14 days.

- Clinical presentation

  o Generalized tetanus

    - Classic symptoms are muscle rigidity and spasms. Typically the first muscles affected are the jaw muscles resulting in *trismus,* or lockjaw, in which the individual is unable to close his or her mouth. The disease progresses to muscles of the face (risus sardonicus), neck, shoulders, and back (opisthotonos). Muscle spasm can be provoked by the slightest stimulation and can be severe enough to threaten ventilation. Dysphagia and autonomic dysfunction can develop.

- o In localized tetanus, muscle spasms occur at or near the site of the wound.

- o In cephalic tetanus, the cranial nerves are affected in association with a wound of the head or neck. Generalized tetanus can follow.

- □ Management: Admittance to ICU under quiet conditions. Wounds should be cleansed properly. The following should be administered: human tetanus immune globulin (TIG) to neutralize unbound toxin; metronidazole to decrease vegetative cells (penicillin G is an alternative) for 10 to 14 days; and immunization against tetanus. Supportive measures include pain medications, antispasmodic agents, and possible ventilator use.

PERTUSSIS

- □ Also known as: Whooping cough

- □ Description: Bacterial infection caused by *Bordetella pertussis.* It is transmitted via aerosolized droplets. The incubation period is usually 7 to 10 days.

- □ Diagnosis: Clinically made. Culture from a nasopharyngeal swab remains the gold standard for diagnosis.

- □ Clinical presentation: The disease has 3 stages:

- o Catarrhal: Nonspecific symptoms of an upper respiratory infection; typically lasts 1 to 2 weeks

- o Paroxysmal: Severity of cough increases; hard coughs followed by a "whoop" on inspiration. Coughing may be hard enough to cause vomiting. Paroxysms can be severe enough to cause hypoxia. This stage typically lasts 2 to 4 weeks

- o Convalescent: Symptoms gradually lessen in severity; this stage may last 2 to 3 weeks.

Cough may persist for months despite resolution of the disease. Pneumonia is a frequent complication.

- □ Management: Treatment is generally supportive. Antibiotics must be given prior to the onset of cough to be effective at treating the infection, although it can still limit the spread to others. Erythromycin is the antibiotic of choice; clarithromycin and azithromycin are alternatives.

ERYTHEMA INFECTIOSUM

☐ Also known as: Fifth disease

☐ Description: Viral infection caused by parvovirus B19. Transmission is via contact with respiratory secretions or contact with blood. Contagiousness is during the prodromal stage; once rash has developed, the patient is no longer infectious. Cases usually occur in late winter and early spring. Incubation period from exposure to onset of symptoms is usually 4 to 14 days.

☐ Diagnosis: The diagnosis is made via detection of serum parvovirus B19-specific IgM levels.

☐ Clinical presentation

　o Flu-like symptoms occur first, lasting 7 to 10 days

　　■ Fever

　　■ Sore throat

　　■ Runny nose

　　■ Headache

　　■ Malaise

　　■ Myalgias

　　■ Arthralgias occur commonly in adults

　o Rash follows often but not always

　　■ First, an erythematous facial rash with a "slapped cheek" appearance occurs

　　■ Second, a generalized, maculopapular, lace-like rash begins on the trunk then spreads to the neck, arms, buttocks, and legs. This rash is often pruritic. It can last up to 7 days. It can come back if the patient is subjected to stress, sun, or increased temperatures.

　o Immunocompromised individuals can develop chronic, transfusion-dependant anemia. In patients who have blood disorders, transient aplastic crisis can develop.

　o Infection during pregnancy can cause hydrops fetalis.

☐ Management: Supportive care

10

DERMATOLOGICAL CONDITIONS

- Acne vulgaris

- Alopecia

- Cutaneous fungal infections

- Hirsutism

- Impetigo

- Melanocytic nevi

- Psoriasis

- Atopic dermatitis

- Seborrheic dermatitis

- Rhus dermatitis

- Contact/allergic dermatitis

- Skin cancer

  - Basal cell carcinoma

  - Squamous cell carcinoma

- Melanoma

- Urticaria and angioedema

Rehberg RS, Rehberg JS.
Cram Session in General Medical Conditions:
A Handbook for Students & Clinicians (pp. 143-156).
© 2012 Taylor & Francis Group.

- Warts

- Cellulitis

- Folliculitis

- Molluscum contagiosum

ACNE VULGARIS

- Also known as: Acne

- Description: Common skin condition of adolescents and young adults. Acne lesions are ultimately the result of the interaction between increased androgenic activity and overgrowth of acne bacteria *Propionibacterium acnes*.

- Clinical presentation

  o Face, chest, and back may be affected

  o Severity of the condition varies

  o Open comedones (blackheads)

  o Closed comedones (whiteheads)

  o Papules

  o Pustules

  o Nodules

  o Scarring

- Management: Patients to be encouraged not to "pick at" lesions, which can increase scarring. Dietary restrictions are not recommended because food has no effect on the development of acne. Treatment initially includes topical antibiotics, benzoyl peroxide washes or gels, and topical retinoids. Oral antibiotics are used with worsening of lesions. For severe acne, isotretinoin and an intralesional steroid injection can be used.

ALOPECIA

- Also known as: Baldness

- Description: Loss of hair. Hair loss disorders are either nonscarring (noncicatricial) or scarring (cicatricial).

  - Nonscarring alopecia can be the result of systemic conditions such as iron-deficiency anemia, thyroid conditions, and systemic lupus erythematosus. There is no evidence of inflammation, skin atrophy, or scarring. Hair loss may be reversible.

    - There are several forms of nonscarring alopecia which are as follows:

      - Androgenetic (pattern) baldness

      - Alopecia areata

      - Drug-induced

      - Chemotherapy-induced

      - Telogen effluvium

    - Causes

      - Termination of pregnancy

      - Oral contraceptive use

      - Stress of surgery

      - High fevers

      - "Crash" dieting can precede telogen effluvium

    - Treatment: Treatment options vary according to the cause. In systemic conditions, control the underlying condition. Intralesional injection of corticosteroids can treat alopecia areata; topical minoxidil may prevent the progression of androgenic baldness. In women, antiandrogens can be used. Hair transplantation can be successful.

  - Scarring alopecia: There is permanent damage or destruction of the hair follicles; this can be due to infection or inflammation. Hair loss is irreversible.

- Causes

  - Infection

  - Neoplasms

  - Developmental defects and hereditary disorders

  - Chemical and physical agents

  - Unknown origin

- Treatment: Diagnose the cause and treat it early to prevent further scarring.

CUTANEOUS FUNGAL INFECTIONS

- Description: Superficial infection with dermatophytes including genera *Trichophyton, Epidermophyton,* and *Microsporum.* Infection is acquired from another person by fomites, from contact with animals such as puppies or cats, or soil. They are classified according to the affected site of the body. Itching may or may not be present.

- Clinical presentation

  - Tinea corporis (ringworm): Found on the neck, trunk, and extremities. Looks like a raised, erythematous ring with a scaly border and central clearing.

  - Tinea cruris (jock itch): Looks like erythematous scaly patches with sharp margins and central clearing in the thighs and groin, usually sparing the scrotum and penis.

  - Tinea pedis (athlete's foot): Often asymptomatic but can present with itching and burning; secondary bacterial infection causes pain. Appears on different locations of the foot.

    - Interdigital: In between toes; erythema, maceration, scaling, and fissuring.

    - Moccasin: Lateral and sole of foot; erythematous, white scaly patches; hyperkeratosis.

    - Ulcerative: Interdigital lesion spreading on to top and sole of foot.

    - Inflammatory/bullous: Sole, instep; erythema, scaling erosion, vesicles, and bullae. Bacterial infection causes pus.

o Tinea manuum: Found on the palms of the hands. Usually associated with tinea pedis. Looks like erythematous, scaling patches; fissuring; hyperkeratosis; papules, grouped vesicles; or pustules with secondary bacterial infection.

o Tinea capitis: Looks like erythematous, scaly patches on the scalp; alopecia may or may not be present.

□ Management: Proper hygiene. Keep area clean and dry; utilize powder containing miconazole or tolnaftate. For macerated lesions, use open, wet compresses with Burrow solution. Topical antifungals include miconazole, clotrimazole, naftifine, tolnaftate, and ciclopiroxalamine and are not for use on the hair. Systemic antifungals can be used for hair and thickened areas of skin and for lesions unresponsive to topical agents. They are used in cases with extensive lesions and include griseofulvin, ketoconazole, itraconazole, and terbinafine.

HIRSUTISM

□ Description: Increased hair growth due to excessive secretion of androgens, such as testosterone

□ Causes

o Polycystic ovary syndrome

o Ovarian tumors

o Adrenal gland defects

o Pituitary tumors

o Medication use

o Idiopathic or familial

□ Clinical presentation

o Increased hair on the upper lip, chin, cheeks, central chest, and abdomen

o Menstrual irregularities

o Acne

o Defeminization

o Virilization: Increased muscularity, acne, clitoral hypertrophy, deepening of the voice, and balding

- Management: Treat the underlying cause

  - Cosmetic: Waxing, shaving, electrolysis, and bleaching unwanted hair

  - Medications: Spironolactone, antiandrogens, oral contraceptives, corticosteroids, and metformin

IMPETIGO

- Description: Superficial skin infection secondary to *Staphylococcus aureus* or group A beta-hemolytic *Streptococcus pyogenes,* or mixed. It is contagious.

- Clinical presentation

  - Usually on exposed skin such as the face and extremities

  - Primary infection occurs at minor skin breaks

  - Secondary infection at sites of pre-existing skin conditions

  - Impetigo can be bullous or nonbullous

    - Small vesicles rupture, becoming erosions covered by honey-colored crusts

    - Bullous impetigo has bullae filled with clear yellow fluid

    - Impetigo resulting in deep ulceration of the skin is called *ecthyma*

- Management: Treat with topical mupirocin ointment. Systemic antibiotics are used in cases of multiple lesions or failure of topical ointment.

MELANOCYTIC NEVI

- Also known as: Moles

- Description: Benign pigmented skin lesions composed of melanocytes. Moles are extremely common and can be found over the entire body. There are numerous types of moles. Some of the more common ones are acquired melanocytic nevi, dermal melanocytic nevocellular nevi, blue nevi, Spitz nevi, halo melanocytic nevi, and dysplastic melanocytic nevi.

- Clinical presentation: Each type of mole presents with different characteristics.

    - Small (< 1.0 cm)

    - Well-circumscribed

    - Uniformly pigmented

    - Macules, papules, or nodules

    - Round, oval, or dome-shaped

    - Smooth or hyperkeratotic

    - Can present with small hairs

    - Colors can be skin-colored, pink, tan, brown, dark brown, black, blue, blue-gray, or blue-black

- Management: In most cases, no treatment is necessary. Moles should be monitored for changes. If atypical features develop, surgical excision is warranted.

PSORIASIS

- Description: A chronic recurrent inflammatory skin disorder. Several variants exist. It may be associated with psoriatic arthritis. Trauma, such as scratching, to pre-existing lesions can precipitate proliferation, or Koebner's phenomenon.

- Clinical presentation

    - Well-marginated, red plaques with silvery-white scales

    - Pitting of the nails

    - Typically, extensor surfaces are affected—elbows and knees; also the scalp, buttocks, hands, soles, and nails

- Management: Cutaneous hydration should be utilized. Treatments include topical glucocorticoid creams or ointments, tar compounds such as tar shampoo, topical retinoids, and UV light therapy. Methotrexate may be used if severe.

ATOPIC DERMATITIS

- ☐ Also known as: Eczema

- ☐ Description: Atopic dermatitis can be acute or subacute, but is usually a chronic inflammation of the epidermis and dermis. It is usually associated with a family or personal history of asthma, allergic rhinitis, or hay fever. A common itch-scratch-rash-itch cycle exists. Exacerbating factors include allergies, emotional stress, infections, irritants, hormonal, seasonally related changes, and clothing.

It can be complicated commonly by *Staphylococcus aureus* leading to erosions and crusting as well as herpes simplex, which leads to eczema herpeticum.

- ☐ Clinical presentation

  - o Severely pruritic

  - o Commonly found on the neck, face, eyelids, wrist, hands, feet, and particularly the antecubital and popliteal fossas

  - o In infants, it is commonly found on the face

  - o Lesions appear as erythematous patches, plaques, and papules

  - o Lichenification (thickening of the skin with increased skin markings)

  - o Fissures

  - o Alopecia (lateral third of the eyebrow)

  - o Periorbital pigmentation secondary to rubbing of eyelids

- ☐ Management: Discourage patients' need to rub or scratch. The key is avoidance of irritants and allergens.

Treatment varies according to the stage of dermatitis and includes hydration via baths or soaks (using oatmeal or saline solutions), the application of wet dressings, emollients, topical corticosteroids of varying potencies according to severity of dermatitis, oral antihistamines, and topical or oral antibiotics (as indicated). In severe cases, phototherapy with UVB, UVB-UVA can be beneficial, as can photochemotherapy with photochemotherapy. Systemic corticosteroids should be avoided except in extensive cases and only used for short course.

SEBORRHEIC DERMATITIS

- Also known as: Dandruff; "cradle cap" in infants
- Description: Chronic dermatosis that can be associated with intense pruritis. Associated with the presence of the yeast *Pityrosporum ovale*
- Clinical presentation
    - Erythematous patches, often with yellowish, greasy, or white dry scaling of varying size
    - Crusting and fissures usually found on scalp, eyebrows, beard, nasolabial folds, trunk, body folds, and genitalia
- Management: Treatments include shampoos containing selenium sulfide, tar, or zinc pyrithione. Two percent ketoconazole cream or shampoo can be used. In severe cases, hydrocortisone or desonide cream is utilized.

RHUS DERMATITIS

- Also known as: Poison ivy, poison sumac, poison oak
- Description: Delayed, cell-mediated hypersensitivity reaction to resin of plants of genus *Rhus*
- Clinical presentation
    - Intensely pruritic
    - Lesions are often linear and present at the site of contact
    - Lesions progress from erythematous papules, to vesicles, to crusting, and lastly, to scaling
- Management: Treatment with topical glucocorticoids. Systemic glucocorticoids are used, if severe.

CONTACT/ALLERGIC DERMATITIS

- Description: Skin reaction caused by contact with exogenous substances. Reactions may be acute or chronic. With contact dermatitis, reactions are the result of frequent exposure to chemicals/irritants such as detergents, soaps, or perfumes. With allergic dermatitis, the reaction is to an antigen: antimicrobials, anesthetics, hair dyes, latex, adhesive tape, or nickel.

- Clinical presentation
  - At the site of exposure:
    - Erythema
    - Vesicles
    - Crusting
    - Scaling
    - Thickened skin
    - Chronic exposure leads to fissures and crusting
- Management: Encourage patients to avoid exposure to irritants or allergens. Localized lesions are treated with topical steroids; for severe or widespread involvement, systemic corticosteroids are utilized. With facial or groin involvement, nonsteroidal ointments are used.

SKIN CANCER

BASAL CELL CARCINOMA

- Description: Basal cell carcinoma (BCC) is the most common type of skin cancer. Tumors can be locally invasive, but metastasis rarely occurs. These lesions occur mostly on sun-exposed skin in light-skinned individuals. Several types with different appearances exist.
- Clinical presentation: BCC are usually papular or nodular and may be umbilicated. They may be shiny, pink, or red in color; translucent or "pearly." Telangiectasias may be present.

SQUAMOUS CELL CARCINOMA

- Description: Squamous cell carcinoma (SCC) is a malignant skin tumor. It can occur on the skin or mucous membranes. Metastasis can occur. SCC can develop as a result of sun exposure. Other etiologies exist including human papillomavirus (HPV), immunosuppression, and exposure to carcinogens such as arsenic or oils.
- Clinical presentation: There are 2 types of squamous cell carcinoma: highly differentiated and poorly differentiated. Each has a distinct appearance. Highly differentiated SCC is an erythematous, hard, indurated papule, nodule, or plaque. It can be round and smooth or exhibit hyperkeratosis and ulcerations. Poorly differentiated SCC is an erythematous, soft, fleshy papule, nodule, or papillomatous vegetation. It may exhibit erosions with an irregular border.

□ Management: BCC and SCC are typically treated by excision of tumor using either standard procedure or Mohs micrographic surgery. Radiation therapy is reserved for use when surgical treatment is difficult, such as with tumors on the face.

MELANOMA

□ Description: Malignant melanoma is the most common cause of death from skin disease and has a high risk potential for metastasis. Fair-skinned, sun-exposed individuals are at risk. Other risk factors include immunosuppression, family history, previous melanoma, and individuals with an increasing number of nevi. Melanoma should be considered with any nevus that has enlarged, changed in appearance, or become itchy, tender, or bloody. Several subtypes of melanoma exist.

□ Clinical presentation: The ABCDEs of melanoma

  o **A**symmetry

  o **B**order irregularity

  o **C**olor variation within a lesion

  o **D**iameter > 6 mm (pencil eraser)

  o **E**nlargement; elevation

□ Clinical presentation of each subtype varies. The American Joint Commission on Cancer has developed a classification system for melanotic tumors. Each stage of classification has a different prognosis for survival.

□ Management: Surgical excision of the lesion with narrow margins is the treatment of choice. If metastasis exists, therapy can include surgical excision, radiation therapy, and/or chemotherapy.

URTICARIA AND ANGIOEDEMA

□ Also known as: Hives

□ Description: A generally self-limiting hypersensitivity reaction lasting 1 to 2 weeks. Urticaria involves the dermis while angioedema involves subcutaneous or submucosal tissue. The reaction may be acute, lasting less than 6 weeks, or chronic, lasting more than 6 weeks.

- Classifications of reaction
  - Immunologic
    - IgE-Dependent: Often atopic; secondary to specific antigens such as foods, medications, or insect bites
    - Complement-mediated: Related to serum sickness or transfusion reaction
  - Nonimmunologic
    - Physical: Dermatographism, delayed-pressure, vibratory, cold urticaria, cholinergic urticaria, or solar urticaria
    - Autoimmune disease: Rheumatic disease such as systemic lupus erythematosus (SLE) or vasculitis
    - Allergic: Drug-induced such as from angiotensin-converting enzyme (ACE)-inhibitors, aspirin, nonsteroidal anti-inflammatory drugs, drugs releasing histamine, or antibiotics; radiocontrast media; or foods containing high level of histamine such as strawberries, shellfish, and cheese
    - Idiopathic
- Clinical presentation
  - Urticaria
    - Transient, circumscribed wheals
    - Raised, erythematous plaques
    - Intensely pruritic
    - Blanches with pressure and may coalesce
  - Angioedema
    - Swelling around the eyes and lips, hands, feet, and genitalia that can be painful and tender to the touch
- Management: Prevention by avoidance of the precipitating factor.
  - Treatment with antihistamines: H_1-receptor blockers, both nonsedating (eg, Claritin) and sedating (eg, Benadryl) and H_2-receptor blockers (eg, Zantac). Leukotriene modifiers and oral prednisone have been used. Tricyclic antidepressants can be given

in chronic cases. Intramuscular injection of epinephrine is given in emergency situations.

WARTS

- Description: Benign hyperkeratotic skin-colored papules with a verrucous (irregular) surface caused by HPV. Warts are found on the skin or mucosal surfaces. Transmission is through skin-to-skin contact or by way of fomites (inanimate objects). Warts usually undergo spontaneous resolution.

- Clinical presentation

  - Common warts (verruca vulgaris)—Firm, hyperkeratotic papules that are typically found on hands, fingers, and knees; characteristic "red dots"

  - Plantar warts (verruca plantaris)—Plaque with rough, thickened skin; plantar foot; characteristic brown-black dots; resemble corns or callouses; can be painful with pressure

  - Flat warts (verruca plana)—Sharply defined, flat papules; typically on face, dorsum of hand, or shins

- Management: Destruction of warts utilizing liquid nitrogen, curettage, laser, light destruction, or acids

CELLULITIS

- Description: Acute, pyogenic infection of the dermis and subcutaneous tissues most commonly found in the lower extremity. Typically caused by *S aureus,* group A beta-hemolytic and *S pyogenes.*

- Clinical presentation

  - Occurs at an already existing break in the skin barrier such as from surgical wounds, trauma, mucosal infection, ulcers, and chronic dermatoses

  - Hot, erythematous, edematous, and tender plaques with a sharply defined border

- Management: Supportive care—immobilization, elevation, and analgesia. Oral antimicrobial therapy is used. Intravenous antibiotics are used in severe cases.

FOLLICULITIS

- ❑ Description: Infection of the hair follicle caused by blockage, friction, rubbing, or damage

- ❑ Clinical presentation: Itching, burning, red papules, and pustules. Commonly occurs on the face, beard, neck, chest, scalp, legs, and buttocks.

- ❑ Management: Several variants exist with specific treatment protocols:

  - o Staphylococcal infection—Mupirocin ointment, oral antibiotics

  - o *Pseudomonas aeruginosa* ("hot tub folliculitis")—Usually resolves spontaneously; ciprofloxacin

  - o Gram-negative folliculitis (associated with treatment of acne)—Discontinue oral antibiotics, wash with benzoyl peroxide

  - o Fungal—Topical antifungals

  - o Viral—Oral antiviral agents

  - o Irritant (oils)—Removal of the substance; use of drying agents

  - o Pseudofolliculitis barbae—Ingrown hairs in the beard area; pustules are near, not in the hair follicles. Treatment includes growing a beard and use of chemical depilatories.

MOLLUSCUM CONTAGIOSUM

- ❑ Description: Benign, self-limiting viral infection of the skin caused by a poxvirus. Spread via direct contact, including sexual contact or by way of fomites. Autoinoculation is possible.

- ❑ Clinical presentation

  - o Umbilicated

  - o Pearly

  - o Dome-shaped papules

  - o Found on the trunk, face, genitalia, and skin folds

- ❑ Management: Spontaneous remission of lesions. Treatment can be utilized to prevent autoinoculation or spread to others including curettage, liquid nitrogen, topical agents, and electrocautery.

11

RHEUMATOLOGICAL CONDITIONS

- ☐ Ankylosing spondylitis
- ☐ Fibromyalgia
- ☐ Gouty arthritis
- ☐ Juvenile rheumatoid arthritis
- ☐ Osteoarthritis
- ☐ Osteoporosis
- ☐ Rheumatoid arthritis
- ☐ Systemic lupus erythematosus

Rehberg RS, Rehberg JS.
Cram Session in General Medical Conditions:
A Handbook for Students & Clinicians (pp. 157-166).
© 2012 Taylor & Francis Group.

ANKYLOSING SPONDYLITIS

☐ Also known as: AS

☐ Description: A form of arthritis, ankylosing spondylitis (AS) is a systematic inflammatory disorder that causes inflammation between spinal joints, or fuses spinal vertebrae and inflames the sacroiliac joints. AS affects more men than women, and strikes 1 in 1,000 people under the age of 40.

☐ Causes: AS is an autoimmune disorder that occurs most commonly in men who have the HLA-B27 gene.

☐ Clinical presentation

o Achilles tendonitis

o Chest pain on inspiration and restriction of lung capacity

o Fatigue

o Kyphosis

o Lack of flexibility

o Lower back pain (sometimes nocturnal)

o Weight loss

☐ Management: The treatment goals focus on pain relief, preventing the loss of joint range of motion, and the protection of the patient's organs. Nonsteroidal anti-inflammatory drugs (NSAIDs) are traditionally used to reduce the pain, decrease joint inflammation, and muscle spasms. Therapeutic exercises should be done with an emphasis on proper posture and joint motion.

FIBROMYALGIA

☐ Also known as: Myofascial pain syndrome, fibrositis, fibromyositis

☐ Description: Fibromyalgia is chronic disorder characterized by widespread and often nonspecific muscle and soft tissue pain and tenderness, among other symptoms. Resulting pain and fatigue can be severe and impact activities of daily living.

☐ Causes: The cause of fibromyalgia is unknown. Factors that may precipitate the condition include previous significant physical or emotional event or injury, repetitive injury, or illness. Other theories regarding cause include genetics and central nervous system abnormalities.

☐ Clinical presentation: Typical areas of pain include the neck, upper back, rib cage, hip, and knees. Symptoms often appear spontaneously.

  o Muscle pain

  o Soft tissue pain

  o Depression

  o Exercise intolerance

  o Fatigue

  o Headache

  o Insomnia

  o Irritable bowel syndrome

  o Mood disturbances

☐ Management: Primary treatment goals include pain relief, stress relief, and sleep quality. Nonopioid analgesics may be prescribed for pain relief. Therapeutic exercise and modalities; stress management may also aid in the management of symptoms.

GOUTY ARTHRITIS

☐ Also known as: Gout

☐ Description: A form of arthritis characterized by the build-up of uric acid, resulting in the deposit of monosodium urate crystals in the joint spaces between the bones. The acute arthritis is initially monoarticular and often involves the first metatarsophalangeal joint or the knee, but it can also attack the wrists, elbows, and ankles.

☐ Causes

  o High levels of uric acid (hyperuricemia) in the blood

  o Genetics

  o Biochemical abnormalities

  o Obesity

- o A diet rich in red meats and organ meat, such as liver

- o Alcohol use (especially beer)

- o Underlying kidney disease

- □ Clinical presentation

  - o Excruciating acute joint pain

  - o Joint tenderness

  - o Warmth

  - o Redness

  - o Joint stiffness

  - o Joint inflammation

  - o Raised bumps at the affected joints ("Tophi")

  - o Intermittent fever

  - o Fatigue

- □ Management: The treatment of the acute gouty attack includes NSAIDs and colchicine. To prevent reoccurring attacks, use of uric acid-lowering medications such as allopurinol should be used daily. There should be a focus on the prevention of further deposition of uric crystals by lowering the patient's serum urate levels through proper medication, proper diet, and adequate fluid intake.

JUVENILE RHEUMATOID ARTHRITIS

- □ Also known as: JRA

- □ Description: A chronic form of arthritis that affects children—usually age 16 or younger—characterized by joint swelling, stiffness, and decreased range of motion

- □ Causes: Juvenile rheumatoid arthritis (JRA) is an autoimmune disorder. The cause of JRA is unknown.

- □ Clinical presentation: Common JRA symptoms include the following:

  - o Joint pain

  - o Inflammation

- o Stiffness

- o Swelling

- o Back pain

- o Decreased range of motion

- o Gait abnormality

- □ Other symptoms may include the following:

  - o Fever

  - o Rash

  - o Swollen lymph nodes

  - o Eye abnormalities (pain, redness, photophobia, and vision difficulties)

- □ Management: The treatment for JRA is similar to adult rheumatoid arthritis. NSAIDs may help reduce the symptoms, and disease-modifying antirheumatic drugs can also be used. Therapeutic exercises and modalities, as well as bracing, splinting, and other supportive measures may also help improve function, minimize unnecessary stress on inflamed joints, and help prevent flexion contractures.

OSTEOARTHRITIS

- □ Also known as: OA, degenerative joint disease, osteoarthrosis, hypertrophic osteoarthritis

- □ Description: OA is an inflammatory joint disease and is classified as either primary or secondary. Primary osteoarthritis results from an unhealthy aging process. It most commonly develops after the age of 45 and affects weight-bearing joints, especially when joints are placed under excessive long-term stress from supporting too much weight or from normal weight demands placed on weak and unhealthy joints. Secondary OA is the less common. It often appears before the age of 40 and is most commonly caused by sudden or reoccurring trauma.

- □ Causes

  - o Cumulative stress placed on joints throughout the lifespan

  - o Biomechanical changes

  - o Diet and food allergies

- o Hormonal imbalance

- o Insulin resistance or deficiency

- o Nutrient deficiencies

- o Obesity

- □ Clinical presentation: Onset is typically gradual, progressing over many years.

  - o Pain

  - o Joint stiffness

  - o Crepitus

  - o Development of bone spurs

  - o Joint effusion

  - o Limited joint mobility

  - o Impaired functionality

- □ Management: Treatment goals are to increase joint strength, maintain or improve joint movement, pain relief, and to reduce the disabling effects of the disease. Treatment can include medications ranging from over-the-counter medications, to NSAIDs, to injectable corticosteroids, or artificial joint fluid. Physical rehabilitation that focuses on exercises for strength, flexibility, endurance, and the education of daily lifestyle modifications can be beneficial to the patient. Adjunctive treatments can include bracing and/or surgery.

OSTEOPOROSIS

- □ Description: Osteoporosis is a progressive metabolic bone disease that decreases bone density and thins bone tissue over time. Bone strength is dependent upon size and density. Bone density is dependent upon levels of calcium, phosphorus, and other minerals. A deficiency in these minerals causes an erosion of structural support within the bone. In women, bone loss can increase dramatically during menopause as a result of lower estrogen levels. Men can also develop osteoporosis due to low levels of estrogen.

- Causes

  - Low estrogen levels

  - Thin build

  - Immobilization

  - Extended sedentary periods

  - Insufficient dietary intake of calcium, phosphate, and vitamin D

  - Cigarette smoking

  - Excessive caffeine or alcohol use

- Clinical presentation

  - Back pain

  - Fractures with little or no trauma

  - Loss of height over time

  - Postural changes such as increased thoracic kyphosis

- Management: The treatment goals for osteoporosis are to preserve bone mass, control pain, prevent fractures, and maintain function. Several treatment possibilities exist including modification of risk factors, medication, identification of possible secondary risk factors that can cause injury (ie, falls due to vision impairment, coordination impairment, or mental confusion), patient education, orthopedic supports, therapeutic and recreational weight-bearing exercise, and diet modification. Regular exercise can reduce the likelihood of bone fractures. Educating patients on how to maintain a diet with the appropriate amounts of calcium, vitamin D, and protein can also be helpful.

RHEUMATOID ARTHRITIS

- Also known as: RA

- Description: RA is an autoimmune disorder that occurs when the patient's own immune system attacks its own body tissues. It is a chronic inflammatory disorder that most typically affects the small joints. RA differs from osteoarthritis in that it affects the lining of the joints, causing a painful swelling that can eventually result in articular structure damage and cause systemic infections. Women are more likely to get RA than men.

- Causes: There are many possible causes to RA occurring in various combinations and to various degrees including the following:

  o Food allergies

  o Nutritional deficiencies

  o Toxicity

  o Intestinal permeability by microorganisms

- Clinical presentation: The onset of RA symptoms is unpredictable. Onset can be slow with mild discomfort in the joints, morning stiffness, and low-grade fevers. Symptoms can develop gradually or rapidly. These symptoms can be debilitating in nature and are shown to occur more commonly in cases with multiple causative factors such as infection, nutritional deficiencies, and toxicity.

- Symptoms of RA may include the following:

  o Anemia

  o Arthritis of 3 or more joints

  o Eye irritation, itching, and discharge

  o Fatigue

  o Limited joint range of motion

  o Loss of appetite

  o Lung inflammation

  o Morning stiffness for 1 hour or more

  o Numbness or tingling

  o Rheumatoid nodules

  o Serum rheumatoid factor

  o Skin redness or inflammation

  o Symmetric arthritis

  o Swollen glands

  o Widespread muscle aches

□ Management: Treatment involves rest, exercise in moderation, proper nutrition, and medication. Additional treatment includes bracing, splinting, proper footwear, and—in some cases—surgery.

SYSTEMIC LUPUS ERYTHEMATOSUS

□ Also known as: SLE, lupus, disseminated lupus erythematosus

□ Description: A chronic multisystem inflammatory disorder (autoimmune disease) that mostly affects young women. Inflammation can affect multiple body systems including blood, joints, kidneys, heart, lungs, and skin. It may occur at any age or race, but appears most often in those aged 10 to 50 years and in African Americans and Asians.

□ Causes: The definitive cause is unknown. It is likely that lupus presents as a result of genetic and environmental factors.

□ Clinical presentation: Most patients present with mild symptoms that worsen and then disappear completely over a period of time. Symptoms include the following:

o Joint pain/arthritis

o Cardiac inflammation including pericarditis, endocarditis, or myocarditis

o Chest pain/discomfort

o Cardiac arrhythmias

o Fatigue/malaise/myalgias

o Fever

o Nausea and vomiting

o Seizures

o Photophobia/visual disturbances

o Swollen glands

o Skin rash—a "butterfly" pattern over the cheeks and bridge of the nose

o Abdominal pain

o Blood disorders/abnormal blood clotting

- o Hematuria

- o Hemoptysis

- o Fingers that change color upon pressure or in the cold

- o Hair loss

- o Mouth sores

- o Epistaxis

- o Parasthesias in the extremities

- o Difficulty swallowing

- □ Management: Treatment for lupus depends on the signs and symptoms, with the primary treatment goal being management of symptoms. Mild disease that involves a rash, headaches, fever, arthritis, pleurisy, and pericarditis requires little therapy. Treatment options may include the use of NSAIDs, corticosteroids, and sun protection (ie, sunscreens and UV clothing). Patients who begin to experience more severe symptoms should be referred to a rheumatologist for proper treatment.

12

PSYCHOLOGICAL CONDITIONS

- □ Anorexia nervosa

- □ Anxiety

- □ Attention deficit/hyperactivity disorder

- □ Binge eating disorder

- □ Bulimia

- □ Depression

- □ Insomnia

- □ Obsessive-compulsive disorder

- □ Seasonal affective disorder

- □ Schizophrenia

Rehberg RS, Rehberg JS.
*Cram Session in General Medical Conditions:
A Handbook for Students & Clinicians* (pp. 167-176).
© 2012 Taylor & Francis Group.

ANOREXIA NERVOSA

☐ Description: Anorexia nervosa is a serious and sometimes chronic eating disorder. Patients with anorexia nervosa obsess about their weight and amount of food they intake. It can result in starvation. The patient typically either refuses to or cannot maintain a normal healthy body weight for his or her age and height. Persons with this condition may be fearful of weight gain and/or obesity, even when they are underweight. The vast majority (95%) of anorexia nervosa cases involve females. Most people with this disorder do not realize that they have a disorder.

☐ Causes: The exact cause of anorexia nervosa is unknown. It is more common in women, particularly young adolescent women. There seems to be a link to high achievers as well the perceived social norms of body appearance.

☐ Clinical presentation

   o Significant weight loss

   o Amenorrhea

   o Hair loss

   o Recurrent overuse injuries

   o Stress fractures

   o Cold extremities

   o Inability to concentrate

   o Compulsive exercise behaviors

   o Low self esteem

   o Poor body image

   o Wearing baggy clothes to hide thinness

   o Nervousness about eating in public

   o Obsession about food intake

   o Forceful regurgitation of the food they have eaten

   o Antisocial or excessive behaviors

   o Diuretic or laxative use

- Management: The management of anorexia nervosa begins with recognizing the signs and symptoms of the patient. Once recognized, measures must be taken to assist the patient with regaining lost body weight. Steps must be taken to improve his or her mental functioning and to prevent the disorder from returning.

ANXIETY

- Also known as: Generalized anxiety disorder (GAD)

- Description: Excessive, exaggerated anxiety with regard to daily activities. Patients affected often fear the worst and worry constantly. The anxiety can eventually dominate the patient's rational thinking and interferes with daily functioning.

- Causes: GAD is a common condition. Many factors can play a part in this condition including stress, behavior, and psychological issues.

- Clinical presentation
  - Difficulty concentrating
  - Excessive worrying
  - Headaches
  - Irritability
  - Muscle tension
  - Restlessness
  - Tiredness
  - Trouble sleeping
  - Unrealistic view of problems

- Management: Patients suspected to have GAD should be referred to a mental health specialist (psychiatrist or psychologist). Medication and cognitive behavioral therapy—which must be supportive in nature and focuses on the patient's problems—are the mainstays of most treatment plans.

ATTENTION DEFICIT/HYPERACTIVITY DISORDER

- Also known as: ADHD

- Description: A disorder highlighted by inattentiveness, impulsivity, overactivity, or a combination of the three. Onset often occurs before the ages of 4 to 7 with the peak age of diagnosis between the ages of 8 to 10.

- Causes: The exact cause of ADHD is unknown. It is believed to be a combination of many factors including genetics, environmental factors, and children who have suffered traumatic brain injuries.

- Clinical presentation: The main signs and symptoms of ADHD are inattention, hyperactivity, and impulsivity.

  o Inattention symptoms include the following:

    - Failure to pay attention to fine details

    - Careless mistakes

    - Failure to sustain interest in tasks

    - Failure to remain focused during personal conversations

    - Inability to follow instructions

    - Difficulty in organizing and completing tasks and activities

    - Forgetfulness, which leads to the loss of items

  o Hyperactivity symptoms include the following:

    - Inability to remain still and attentive

    - Inability to act appropriately as the situation dictates

    - Difficulty in playing quietly

  o Impulsivity symptoms including the following:

    - Difficulty waiting his or her turn

    - Patient interrupts or intrudes others

    - Will shout out answers without being called upon

- Management: Goals must be set for management, including a combination of medication and therapy. If the course of treatment is not effective, re-evaluation is necessary. Treatment should include all members of the patient's "team" (teachers, student, and parents).

BINGE EATING DISORDER

- ☐ Description: An eating disorder characterized by frequent consumption of unusually large quantities of food, usually done in secret. Binge eating disorder is considered by some to be the most common eating disorder.

- ☐ Causes: Binge eating disorder is believed to be caused by an underlying psychological food addiction. The disorder may also be of biological origin caused by abnormalities in the hypothalamus.

- ☐ Clinical presentation

  - ○ Frequent episodes of uncontrolled binge eating, often in secret

  - ○ Normal eating in public or social settings, followed by gorging in private

  - ○ Feelings of guilt, depression, or disgust following the binge episode

  - ○ No attempts to reverse the effects of the binge episode, such as vomiting, exercising, or fasting

- ☐ Management: Binge eating disorder is commonly treated through cognitive or behavioral therapy as well as nutritional counseling.

BULIMIA

- ☐ Description: An illness in which a person binges on food, followed by various methods to reverse the effects of the binge eating (ie, purging), commonly through vomiting or the use of laxatives. Bulimia is more common in women than in men and is most common in adolescents.

- ☐ Causes: The exact cause is unknown. However, genetic, psychological, social, and cultural factors are believed to play a role.

- ☐ Clinical presentation

  - ○ Binge eating, followed by remorse and attempts to purge

  - ○ Abuse of laxatives or diuretics

  - ○ Dental cavities and/or erosion of tooth enamel due to vomiting

  - ○ Frequent weighing

  - ○ Gingivitis

    o Halitosis

    o Self-induced vomiting

- Management: Support groups, cognitive-behavioral therapy, and nutritional counseling are therapies that are often used in the treatment of bulimia. In severe cases, drugs may be prescribed to address depression.

DEPRESSION

- Description: The term *depression* can refer to any of a variety of depressive disorders. Depressive disorders can occur at any age. Patients with depressive disorders experience bouts of sadness that may be either severe enough or may occur frequently enough that they begin to effect a person's functional ability. Those affected may become disinterested or can no longer find pleasure from otherwise enjoyable activities.

- Causes: Chemical imbalances in the brain may be a factor; these imbalances may be caused by heredity or triggered by stressful events in a patient's life. It is not uncommon for women to suffer depression after childbirth, a condition known as postpartum depression.

- Clinical presentation: Depression can cause a multitude of problems.

    o Becoming dysfunctional; struggling with concentrating

    o Questioning worthiness

    o Experiencing sleep disorders and fatigue

    o Loss of sexual desire

    o Menstrual problems in females

    o Anxiety

    o Irritability

    o Panic attacks

    o Change in appetite

    o Possible alcohol abuse

    o Suicidal thoughts

- Management: Management of depression most commonly includes a combination of medication and professional counseling. With the proper treatment, patients with depression will improve.

INSOMNIA

- Description: Difficulty in getting to sleep or continuing to stay asleep. It can also be the inability to get a quality night of sleep. Clinical diagnosis of insomnia involves symptoms lasting for greater than 1 month.

- Causes

  - Alcohol

  - Anxiety

  - High caffeine intake

  - Depression

  - Stress

- Clinical presentation

  - Difficulty falling asleep

  - Fatigue

  - Desire to sleep during the day

  - Constant feeling of not sleeping enough

  - Waking up several times during sleep

- Management: The goal of insomnia treatment is to get the patient to develop good sleeping habits. Recommend that the patient do something relaxing 30 minutes prior to going to sleep (this activity will vary on the patient). Other tips can also be provided to help improve sleep quality including avoiding caffeine, alcohol, or nicotine prior to sleep; avoiding daytime naps; and eating and exercising regularly. One should try to develop a bedtime routine which includes both the same location (bed) and time (same time every night) daily.

OBSESSIVE-COMPULSIVE DISORDER

- Also known as: OCD

- Description: An anxiety disorder characterized by unwanted thoughts (obsessions) and/or repetitive behaviors (compulsions). OCD obsessions are typically nonsensical ideas, thoughts, or images. OCD compulsions are behaviors performed repetitively as a means to prevent or reduce anxiety related to the patient's obsessions.

- Causes: The cause of OCD is not known. There are a few theories that exist, including genetics, body chemistry, environmental factors, and insufficient levels of serotonin in the brain.

- Clinical presentation

  o Obsessions can sometimes be theme-oriented.

    - Fear of nonliving things or objects

    - Obsession with keeping things neat and in order

    - Having impulses aggressive in nature

    - Sexual thoughts or images

  o Compulsions are also theme-oriented and may include the following:

    - Counting

    - Checking and rechecking

    - Demanding reassurances

    - Performing repetitive actions

    - Maintaining order

    - Repetitive washing and cleaning

- Management: OCD treatment consists of psychotherapy and pharmacotherapy. Treatment may last a lifetime and may only be able to control symptoms but not necessarily cure the disorder.

SEASONAL AFFECTIVE DISORDER

- Also known as: SAD

- Description: SAD is a type of depression predicated by seasonal patterns. SAD is more commonly seen in the autumn and winter. The disorder tends to occur in climates of long, cold winters or frequent rain or cloudy conditions.

- Causes: The specific cause of SAD is unknown. Possible causes that may affect a person who has SAD include age, the body chemical makeup, and genetics.

- Clinical presentation: The symptoms of SAD depend on the seasons in which a person is affected by the disorder.

- o Symptoms of winter SAD include the following:
    - Appetite changes
    - Anxiety
    - Concentration problems
    - Depression
    - Fatigue
    - Hopelessness
    - Loss of interest
    - Social withdrawal
    - Weight gain
- o Symptoms of spring and summer SAD include the following:
    - Agitation
    - Appetite
    - Anxiety
    - Increased sex drive
    - Irritability
    - Trouble sleeping
    - Weight loss
- ☐ Management: Treatment for SAD may include light therapy, medications, and psychotherapy.

SCHIZOPHRENIA

- ☐ Description: Schizophrenia is a mental disorder in which the patient has difficulty differentiating between reality and fiction. The schizophrenic patient may lose the ability think logically, have abnormal emotional responses, and behave abnormally in social situations.

- ☐ Causes: Schizophrenia is a complex mental disorder and it seems that genetics may be the main underlying cause. An imbalance in the chemical reactions of the brain involving the neurotransmitters dopamine and glutamate—and possibly others—is also a factor.

- Clinical presentation: Schizophrenia is a chronic illness in which a variety of symptoms may be present. Symptoms usually begin in the teenage years or in early adulthood, and develop slowly over the course of months or years.

  o Initial symptoms

    - Concentration problems

    - Feeling isolated

    - Sleeping issues

    - Social withdrawal

  o As the disorder progresses additional symptoms may develop.

    - Delusions

    - Disorganized speech or behaviors

    - Hallucinations

    - Inability to comprehend reality

    - Impaired problem solving

    - Restricted ranges of emotion

- Management: Schizophrenia can be a difficult disorder to treat. During a schizophrenic attack, it may be best to have the patient hospitalized for his or her own protection and basic needs. Medications can change the balance of chemicals in the brain and help control symptoms. In addition, problem-focused forms of therapy and social skills training may be helpful in improving the patient's social functioning and overall improvement. It should be a goal of treatment to provide family support and education because it has been shown that it can be beneficial to both the patient and his or her family.

13

OPHTHALMOLOGICAL CONDITIONS

- ☐ Chalazion

- ☐ Hordeolum

- ☐ Blepharitis

- ☐ Conjunctivitis

- ☐ Myopia

- ☐ Astigmatism

- ☐ Hyperopia

- ☐ Glaucoma

Rehberg RS, Rehberg JS.
Cram Session in General Medical Conditions:
A Handbook for Students & Clinicians (pp. 177-182).
© 2012 Taylor & Francis Group.

CHALAZION

- □ Description: A chronic granulomatous inflammation of a meibomian gland of the eyelid
- □ Clinical presentation
  - o Discomfort in the eyelid
  - o Redness and lump on the inner surface of the eyelid
  - o Vision may be distorted if the chalazion is large enough to press on the cornea
- □ Management: Warm compress. Antibiotics are not indicated. Local incision to remove the chalazion may be required.

HORDEOLUM

- □ Also known as: Stye
- □ Description: Infection of the sebaceous glands of the eyelid, usually caused by *Staphylococcus*
- □ Clinical presentation
  - o Pain
  - o Redness
  - o Swelling
  - o Warmth
- □ Management: Warm compress and topical antibiotics; may require incision and drainage

BLEPHARITIS

- □ Description: Inflammation or infection of the eyelids' margins. Cause may be seborrheic, staphylococcal, or both
- □ Clinical presentation
  - o Redness
  - o Itching

- o Irritation

- o Crusting

- o Small ulcerative lesions in staphylococcal infection

- o Dry scaling along eyelashes; eyelashes may fall out

- o Seborrheic blepharitis has oily scaling; usually associated with seborrhea of the scalp

- □ Management: Topical antibiotic ointment in staphylococcal blepharitis. For seborrheic blepharitis, gently massage the eyelid margin with baby shampoo.

CONJUNCTIVITIS

- □ Also known as: Pink eye

- □ Description: Inflammation of the conjunctiva (lining of the eyelid and eye surface). Causes are varied and usually benign: viral, bacterial, allergic, or can be caused by chemical exposure. Infection is easily passed from one individual to another.

- □ Clinical presentation

- o Itching

- o Burning

- o Red eye

- o Discharge can be watery (viral), purulent (bacterial), or thin/stringy (allergic)

- o Sensation of the eye having something in it

- o Eyelids may be swollen and stuck together upon waking

- o Viral conjunctivitis is often associated with an upper respiratory infection and preauricular adenopathy

- □ Management: Viral conjunctivitis is self-limiting and treated symptomatically. Bacterial conjunctivitis is treated with antibiotic drops or ointment. Antihistamine drops can be used for allergic conjunctivitis. For chemical conjunctivitis, the offending agent should be removed.

MYOPIA

- □ Also known as: Nearsightedness

- □ Description: Difficulty seeing far objects; ability to see near objects clearly. Light rays are not focused on the retina, but in front of it. This is due to either an elongated eyeball or having a cornea with an increased curvature.

- □ Clinical presentation

  - o Headache

  - o Eye squinting when looking at objects in the distance.

- □ Management: Glasses and contact lenses are commonly used. Refractive surgery, such as laser-assisted in situ keratomileusis (LASIK) can be used to correct nearsightedness.

ASTIGMATISM

- □ Description: Partial blurring of an image at any distance. The cornea is irregularly curved; light rays are not uniformly focused on the retina.

- □ Clinical presentation

  - o Headache

  - o Eye strain

- □ Management: Corrective lenses are used.

HYPEROPIA

- □ Also known as: Farsightedness

- □ Clinical presentation: Difficulty seeing near objects; ability to see far objects clearly. Light rays are focused behind the retina due to the irregular shape of the cornea.

- □ Management: Glasses or contact lenses can be used. Refractive surgery can be performed to correct vision.

GLAUCOMA

- Description: Condition of the eye in which increased intraocular pressure causes damage to the optic nerve. If left untreated, permanent vision loss can develop. Glaucoma is subdivided into open-angle glaucoma and angle-closure glaucoma. Open-angle glaucoma is a chronic condition that can develop over months or years. Risk factors include increasing age, African-American race, and family history of glaucoma. Angle-closure glaucoma is typically an acute condition. It is associated with dilation of the pupil, as can occur in dark rooms, when medically induced for ophthalmologic exam, or from anxiety.

- Clinical presentation

  - Open-angle glaucoma

    - Typically asymptomatic in the early stages of the condition

    - Ophthalmologic examination will reveal changes

    - Loss of vision is gradual and first occurs in the periphery

  - Angle-closure glaucoma

    - Extreme pain

    - Blurred vision

    - Halos around lights

    - Red eye

    - Nausea and vomiting

- Management: Routine eye screening is recommended every 2 to 4 years for individuals over 40 years of age. Individuals with risk factors should begin screening after age 30. Screening should be every 1 to 2 years after age 65. Open-angle glaucoma is initially treated with topical agents. Laser therapy and surgery may be necessary. Acute angle-closure glaucoma is a medical emergency. Treatment includes medications, laser therapy, and surgery.

BIBLIOGRAPHY

Bates LS, Szilagyi PG. *Bates' Guide to Physical Examination and History Taking.* 9th ed. Philadelphia, PA: Lippincott Williams & Wilkins; 2005.

Bope ET, Rakel RE, Kellerman RD, eds. *Conn's Current Therapy 2010.* Philadelphia, PA: W. B. Saunders Co; 2010.

DeGowin RL, Brown DD. *DeGowin's Diagnostic Examination.* 7th ed. New York, NY: McGraw-Hill; 2000.

Gould BE. *Pathophysiology for the Health Related Professions.* 2nd ed. Philadelphia, PA: W. B. Saunders Co; 2002.

Libby P, Bonow RO, Mann DL, Zipes DP. *Braunwald's Heart Disease: A Textbook of Cardiovascular Medicine.* 8th ed. Philadelphia, PA: W. B. Saunders Co; 2009.

McPhee SJ, Papadakis MA, Tierney LM, eds. *Current Medical Diagnosis and Treatment.* Los Altos, CA: Lange Medical Publications; 2007.

O'Connor DP, Fincher AL. *Clinical Pathology for Athletic Trainers: Recognizing Systemic Disease.* 2nd ed. Thorofare, NJ: Slack Incorporated; 2008.

Pickering LK, Baker CJ, Long SS, eds. *Red Book: 2006 Report of the Committee on Infectious Diseases.* 27th ed. Elk Grove, IL: American Academy of Pediatrics; 2006.

Porter RS, Kaplan JL, eds. *The Merck Manual of Diagnosis and Therapy.* 19th ed. Rahway, NJ: Merck Research Laboratories; 2011.

Porth C. *Pathophysiology: Concepts of Altered Health States.* Philadelphia, PA: Lippincott, Williams & Wilkins; 2005.

Venes D, Thomas CL, Taber CW, eds. *Taber's Cyclopedic Medical Dictionary.* 19th ed. Philadelphia, PA: F.A. Davis Company; 2001.

INDEX

.

Printed in the United States
by Baker & Taylor Publisher Services